Palliative Practices A-Z

FROM

for the Bedside Clinician

Edited by

Kim K. Kuebler, MN, RN, ANP-CS,
and Peg Esper, MSN, RN, CS, AOCN®

Oncology Nursing Society
Pittsburgh, PA

ONS Publishing Division
Publisher: Leonard Mafrica, MBA, CAE
Director, Commercial Publishing: Barbara Sigler, RN, MNEd
Technical Editor: Dorothy Mayernik, RN, MSN
Senior Staff Editor: Lisa M. George
Copy Editors: Toni Murray, Lori Wilson
Creative Services Assistant: Dany Sjoen

Palliative Practices From A–Z for the Bedside Clinician
Copyright © 2002 by the Oncology Nursing Society

First printing, April 2002
Second printing, June 2006

Library of Congress Control Number: 2002104423
ISBN 1-890504-28-9

Publisher's Note

This book is published by the Oncology Nursing Society (ONS). ONS neither represents nor guarantees that the practices described herein will, if followed, ensure safe and effective patient care. The recommendations contained in this book reflect ONS's judgment regarding the state of general knowledge and practice in the field as of the date of publication. The recommendations may not be appropriate for use in all circumstances. Those who use this book should make their own determinations regarding specific safe and appropriate patient-care practices, taking into account the personnel, equipment, and practices available at the hospital or other facility at which they are located. The editors and publisher cannot be held responsible for any liability incurred as a consequence from the use or application of any of the contents of this book. Figures and tables are used as examples only. They are not meant to be all-inclusive, nor do they represent endorsement of any particular institution by ONS. Mention of specific products and opinions related to those products do not indicate or imply endorsement by ONS.

ONS publications are originally published in English. Permission has been granted by the ONS Board of Directors for foreign translation. (Individual tables and figures that are reprinted or adapted require additional permission from the original source.) However, because translations from English may not always be accurate and precise, ONS disclaims any responsibility for inaccurate translations. Readers relying on precise information should check the original English version.

Printed in the United States of America

Oncology Nursing Society
Integrity • Innovation • Stewardship • Advocacy • Excellence • Inclusiveness

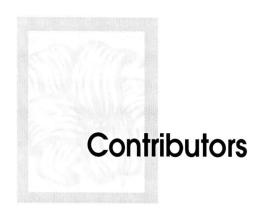

Contributors

Co-Editors

Kim K. Kuebler, MN, RN, ANP-CS
Primary/Oncology/Palliative Care
Adjuvant Therapies, Inc.
Private Practice
Lake, MI
*Agitation, Asthenia, Bereavement,
Caregiver Burden, Dehydration,
Appendix C: Internet Resources,
Glossary*

Peg Esper, MSN, RN, CS, AOCN®
Nurse Practitioner, Medical Oncology
University of Michigan Comprehen-
sive Cancer Center
Ann Arbor, MI
*Anemia; Anorexia, Cachexia, and
Nutritional Support; Infection;
Insomnia; Lymphedema; Pain;
Pruritus; Quality of Life; Urinary
Elimination; Xerostomia; Zoster*

Authors

Costantino Benedetti, MD
Director, Cancer Pain and Palliative
   Medicine Program
Professor, Clinical Anesthesiology
The Ohio State University Arthur G.
   James Cancer Hospital and Richard
   J. Solove Research Institute
Columbus, OH
*Pain, Appendix A: Management of
Neuropathic Pain*

Lynn Borstelmann, RN, MN, CHPN,
   AOCN®
Director, Continuum of Care
University Hospital/SUNY Upstate
   Medical University
Syracuse, NY
Home or Hospital?, Hope, Insurance

William Breitbart, MD
Chief, Psychiatry Service
Department of Psychiatry and
   Behavioral Sciences
Attending Psychiatrist
Pain and Palliative Care Service
Department of Neurology
Memorial Sloan-Kettering Cancer
   Center
New York, NY
Professor of Psychiatry
Department of Psychiatry
Weill College of Medicine of Cornell
   University
Ithaca, NY
Depression

Beth Cohen, RNC, ARNP, MSN
Clinical Nurse Specialist for Medicine
and Surgery
North Broward Hospital District
Ft. Lauderdale, FL
*Cough, Diarrhea, Fatigue, Fever,
Sexuality, Travel*

Jerre Cory, MA, CSW
Executive Director
Nation's Children's Bereavement
Services
East Lansing, MI
*Bereavement, Caregiver Burden,
Funeral Planning, Grief*

Joshua M. Cox, RPh
Board of Directors
Ohio Pain Initiative
Beavercreek, OH
*Depression, Pain, Appendix A:
Management of Neuropathic Pain*

Mellar Davis, MD, FCCP
Medical Director
The Harry R. Horvitz Center for
Palliative Medicine
Taussig Cancer Center
Cleveland Clinic Foundation
Cleveland, OH
*Depression, Nausea and Vomiting,
Pain, Appendix A: Management of
Neuropathic Pain*

Rev. James M. Deshotels, SJ, APRN
Director, Marillac Center for Commu-
nity Health Resources
Daughters of Charity Services of New
Orleans
New Orleans, LA
*Cultural Awareness, Fear, Isolation,
Spirituality*

E. Duke Dickerson, MSc, PhD
Fellow*, Oxford International Centre
for Palliative Care

Oxford, United Kingdom
*Fellowship is funded by Boehringer
Ingelheim
*Depression, Pain, Appendix A:
Management of Neuropathic Pain*

Suzanne W. Dixon, MPH, MS, RD
Director of Outpatient Oncology
Nutrition Services
Oncology Nutrition Specialist and
Epidemiologist
University of Michigan Comprehen-
sive Cancer Center
Ann Arbor, MI
*Anorexia, Cachexia, and Nutri-
tional Support*

Nancy K. English, PhD, APN, CS
Coordinator, Palliative Care
The Children's Hospital
Grant Faculty, Palliative Care Nursing
University of Colorado, School of
Nursing
Denver, CO
Complementary Therapies

Debra E. Heidrich, RN, MSN, CHPN,
AOCN®
Nursing Consultant
West Chester, OH
*Ascites, Death and Dying, Edema,
Skin Lesions*

Jeffery P. Henderson, MS
PhD Program in Counseling Psychol-
ogy
Tennessee State University
Nashville, TN
Depression

Susanne F. Homant, MBA, Doctoral
Candidate
Executive Director
Florida Hospices and Palliative Care
Tallahassee, FL
Hospice Care

Helen K. McHale, MSN, RN, CIIPN
Palliative Care Consultant and Author
Bartlesville, OK
Palliative Care, Terminal Sedation

Marco Pappagallo, MD
Director, Comprehensive Pain
  Treatment Center
Hospital for Joint Diseases—Orthope-
  dic Institute
New York, NY
Associate Professor of Neurology
New York University, School of
  Medicine
*Pain, Appendix A: Management of
Neuropathic Pain*

Martin Perz, JD
Attorney at Law
North Huntingdon, PA
Legal Issues in Pain Management

John L. Shuster, Jr., MD
Director, UAB Center for Palliative
  Care
Associate Professor of Psychiatry and
  Medicine
University of Alabama School of
  Medicine
Birmingham, AL
Depression

Howard Smith, MD
Director of Cancer Pain
Beth Israel Deaconess Medical Center
Harvard Medical School
Boston, MA
*Agitation, Asthenia, Delirium/Acute
Confusion*

Pamela Spencer, BA, MSN, BSN, FNP
Nurse Practitioner
Saginaw Veterans Administration
Saginaw, MI
*Anxiety, Bowel Obstruction,
Dysphagia, Dyspnea*

Karen J. Stanley, RN, MSN, AOCN®,
  FAAN
Nursing Consultant, Palliative Care
Claremont, CA
*Communication, Family Issues,
Psychologic Support*

Carol Taylor, CSFN, RN, PhD
Director, Center for Clinical Bioethics
Assistant Professor, School of Nursing
  and Health Studies
Georgetown University
Washington, DC
*Advance Directives, Ethics,
Appendix B: Advocacy Competen-
cies*

James Varga, RPh, MBA
Director
Pain and Palliative Care Association
  LLC
Orlando, FL
*Pain, Appendix A: Management of
Neuropathic Pain*

Kimberly A. Zielke, MD
Medical Director
MidMichigan VNA/Hospice
Midland, MI
Constipation, Hiccups, Seizures

Contents

Foreword ix
Preface xi
Acknowledgments xiii

Advance Directives 1
Agitation 5
Anemia 9
Anorexia, Cachexia, and Nutritional Support 13
Anxiety 23
Ascites 27
Asthenia 31
Bereavement 35
Bowel Obstruction 39
Caregiver Burden 43
Communication 47
Complementary Therapies 51
Constipation 59
Cough 63
Cultural Awareness 67
Death and Dying 71
Dehydration 77
Delirium/Acute Confusion 81
Depression 85
Diarrhea 89
Dysphagia 93
Dyspnea 97
Edema 101
Ethics 105
Family Issues 111
Fatigue 115

Fear 119
Fever 123
Funeral Planning 127
Grief 129
Hiccups 133
Home or Hospital? 137
Hope 143
Hospice Care 147
Infection 151
Insomnia 155
Insurance 159
Isolation 165
Legal Issues in Pain Management 169
Lymphedema 175
Nausea and Vomiting 179
Pain 185
Palliative Care 193
Pruritus 199
Psychologic Support 203
Quality of Life 207
Seizures 211
Sexuality 215
Skin Lesions 221
Spirituality 227
Terminal Sedation 231
Travel 235
Urinary Elimination 239
Xerostomia 243
Zoster 245

Appendix A: Management of Neuropathic Pain 247
Appendix B: Advocacy Competencies 255
Appendix C: Internet Resources 257
Pharmaceutical Agents Used in This Text 259
Glossary 265
Index 271

Foreword

Modern palliative care developed during the 1960s in the United Kingdom, as a response to the unmet needs of terminally ill patients and their families. This initially British movement soon became global, and a large number of clinical programs emerged around the world.

The assessment and management of the main physical and psychosocial problems of patients, family support, and bereavement counseling were performed for many years with very limited evidence backing up the interventions. This was mostly due to the limited connection between the community-based palliative care programs and the academic institutions and also because of the overwhelming clinical workload on healthcare professionals in these programs.

Fortunately, within the last five years, palliative care has been progressively recognized as a genuine academic pursuit for healthcare professionals in medicine, nursing, psychology, social work, and related professions. As a consequence, a number of teachers and scholars in this area have started to devote a considerable portion of their time to academic activities related to palliative care and end of life. This increased emphasis has increased the body of knowledge significantly and generated much better evidence to guide clinical decision making and daily practice. One of the challenges is how to reach clinicians with this wealth of information.

This book provides an original and highly effective way of providing evidence-based palliative care information to nurses and other healthcare professionals. The authors have made an effort to provide up-to-date information about clinical management, as well as a better understanding of the problems discussed in this book, by describing the etiology and pathophysiology of most of the conditions. The A–Z approach is of great value because it allows busy clinicians easy access to information they need. This book's format will make the book a regular feature in inpatient and outpatient settings where palliative care is regularly delivered.

I would like to congratulate the authors on this excellent contribution. It will increase patient and family access to excellent palliative care, and it also is a reminder for us of how much progress our discipline has made during the last decade.

Eduardo Bruera, MD
Professor and Chair
Department of Symptom Control
and Palliative Care
The University of Texas
M.D. Anderson Cancer Center
Houston, TX

Preface

The need to better understand palliative care is not just for those who choose to work in this field. All healthcare professionals will likely encounter patients living with or dying from advanced illness. This book is a result of the efforts of two advanced practice nurses who believe in the importance of an easy-to-use text on palliative care for healthcare providers. We were fortunate to have expert contributors join us in this endeavor. Our hope is that this book will help to make a difference in the care of individuals at the end of life. We would welcome any comments or suggestions from those of you who have the opportunity to use it in your practice.

Kim K. Kuebler, MN, RN, ANP-CS
Peg Esper, MSN, RN, CS, AOCN®

Acknowledgments

The commitment to improve the quality of life and death comes from all of those who have taught me to do what was right for them. To my beautiful children, Kayne and Kendal, and to both of my parents for their unconditional love and support.

Kim K. Kuebler, MN, RN, ANP-CS

I would like to dedicate this book to my best friend and husband, Jerry, who has always supported me in every endeavor; to my daughter, Melissa; and to my son, Tim. They embody the joy of life. I also am grateful to my patients, who teach me more each day about the need for quality palliative care.

Peg Esper, MSN, RN, CS, AOCN®

Advance Directives

Carol Taylor, CSFN, RN, PhD

Definition

An *advance directive* is a written document that informs healthcare providers of their medical management requests in the event they are unable to do so themselves. A *living will* provides specific instructions about the kinds of health care that should be provided or forgone in particular situations. A *durable power of attorney for health care* appoints an agent the person trusts to make decisions in the event of the appointing person's subsequent incapacity.

Specific Issues Related to Palliative Care

Many families relate narratives of their loved ones' dying being needlessly prolonged by undesired treatment or being hastened when treatment is withheld or withdrawn. Advances in knowledge and technology have proliferated treatment options and complicated healthcare decision making for many conditions. Even when there is a strong consensus about the therapeutic regimen, aggressive treatment options generally are recognized and accepted. The value placed on physical well-being, life goals, the adequacy of resources (financial and human), religious convictions, and cultural values are just some of the factors influencing both patient and caregiver decision making. What is certain is that it is never safe to assume that a patient will prefer the same therapeutic course as the treating clinician.

Patients realistically fear that they will lose control of decision making. It is not uncommon for a patient's voice to be stifled or ignored when a patient wants aggressive therapy withheld or discontinued or when a patient demands aggressive life-sustaining therapy that a clinician judges to be medically futile. Factors contributing to physician reluctance to withhold or withdraw life-sustaining therapy include lack of familiarity with ethical and legal guidelines for withholding and withdrawing medical treatment, misunderstandings about the legal consequences of withholding or withdrawing treatment, failure to embrace preparation for a comfortable and dignified death as a legitimate aim of medicine, and a general lack of ease in initiating discussions about the plan of care as a patient's condition declines.

A. Support for advance care planning (Emanuel, von Gunten, & Ferris, 1999): Common law, federal and state legislation, and official policies of medical organizations support advance care planning.
   1. U.S. Supreme Court, 1990: Upheld the patient's right to self-determination, establishing that the right applies even to patients who are no longer able to direct their own health care, and that decisions for incompetent patients should be based on their previously stated wishes.
   2. Federal law, 1991: The Patient Self-Determination Act (PSDA) requires that patients be informed of their rights to accept or refuse medical treatment and to specify, in advance, the care they would like to receive should they become incapacitated.
   3. State law: The patient's right to specify wishes in advance has been codified into statute in all 50 states. Statutory documents recognized by law include the living will and the durable power of attorney for health care.
   4. Statutory documents are those that are specifically described and defined in state statutes. These documents are to help protect clinicians who honor a patient's wishes. When such documents are used, rights, obligations, and protections are clearly defined.
   5. Nonstatutory or advisory documents are legal. They are based on common law rights. They are supposed to accurately reflect a patient's wishes. In some states or settings, an advisory document is enough; in others, a statutory form should be used as well. In some states, a legal guardian may be necessary if no statutory power of attorney exists for health care.
   6. Professional policy
      a) In 1997, the American Medical Association's Council on Ethical and Judicial Affairs identified advance care planning as an essential component of standard medical practice. It called for physicians to conduct advance planning discussions on a routine basis, using advisory documents as an adjunct to statutory documents, such as the living will and the durable power of attorney for health care. The American College of Physicians' *Ethics Manual,* 4th edition, also supports advance care planning.
      b) The American Nurses Association (ANA) has a position statement on nursing and the PSDA. The ANA position is that "nurses should play a primary role in implementation of the Patient Self-Determination Act (PSDA). It is the responsibility of nurses to facilitate informed decision making for patients making choices about end-of-life care. The nurse's role in education, research, patient care, and advocacy is critical to implementation of the PSDA within all health care settings" (November 18, 1991).

B. Explanations for the failure of many to execute advance directives
   1. Drafting an advance directive means admitting our mortality; this is an uncomfortable subject for many in our death-denying culture.

2. Caregivers wait for patients to initiate conversation about advance directives, and patients wait for caregivers to initiate these discussions.
3. Everyone is "too busy" to have these conversations, and advance care planning does not have an ICD-9 code.
4. Many people fear that the mere existence of an advance directive will prejudice healthcare professionals to withhold desired care.

Strategies to Promote Use of Advance Directives

A. Educate the public and healthcare professionals about advance directives.

B. Incorporate advance care planning into everyday caregiving.

C. Make advance directives a part of the medical record, and ensure that everyone (this includes the patient's surrogate[s] and family) understands the implications for treatment and care (AHA, 1991).

D. Presume nothing about an advance directive until you have read it carefully. Patient preferences can vary widely.

E. Resolve implementation problems.
   1. Conflicts about when an advance directive becomes operative
   2. Conflicts when an attending clinician elects to ignore advance directives
   3. Conflicts when designated surrogates ignore patient preferences documented in an advance directive
   4. Conflicts about how to interpret the content of the directive

Patient Outcomes

A. A documented record exists of the patient's preferences for end-of-life care and identification of the person the patient trusts to make his or her decisions should the patient lack decision-making capacity.

B. Documented patient preferences dictate end-of-life treatment and care when the patient is no longer able to communicate his or her preferences.

Professional Competencies

A. Advance care planning is used to identify and document the patient's preferences for end-of-life care.

B. Advance directives are modified and reviewed when changes in the patient's condition or prognosis ensue.

C. Determinations are made about when an advance directive becomes operative (conditions may vary from state to state).

D. Information is available within the patient's medical record that identifies contact information for the person(s) responsible to make medical decisions for the patient.

E. When the surrogate of a patient who lacks decision-making capacity reports the existence of an advance directive, the healthcare professional obtains copies of the directive, communicates the content of the directive, and, if necessary, facilitates the resolution of conflicts about how the directive is to be determined.

Resources

Advance directives may be obtained from the following sources.

A. Aging With Dignity: www.agingwithdignity.org

B. Choice in Dying: www.choices.org

C. Emanuel, L.L. (1993). Advance directives: What have we learned so far? *Journal of Clinical Ethics, 4,* 8–16.

D. Pearlman, R., Starks, H., Cain, K., Cole, W., Rosengren, D., & Patrick, D. (1992). *Your life choices, planning for future medical decisions: How to prepare a personalized living will.* Seattle, WA: Patient Decisions Support (www.patientdecisions.com).

References

American Hospital Association. (1991). *Put it in writing: A guide to promoting advance directives.* Chicago: Author.

Emanuel, L.L., von Gunten, C.F., & Ferris, F.D. (1999). *The Education for Physicians on End-of-Life Care* (EPEC) *Curriculum.* Princeton, NJ: The Robert Wood Johnson Foundation.

Patient Self-Determination Act of 1990, H.R.5835 [OBRA 1990], 101st Congress (1990).

Agitation

Howard Smith, MD, and Kim K. Kuebler, MN, RN, ANP-CS

Definition

Agitation has been used to describe behaviors, syndromes, and outcomes of multiple psychiatric or medical problems. Agitation can include a group of symptoms involving several underlying disorders. Nonspecific agitation also may be a result of psychotic illness, a personality disorder, an amnesic disorder, anger, fear, irritation, or interpersonal conflict that often is the result of unfinished business (Kuebler & Heidrich, 2001). Agitation is synonymous with restlessness and is very prevalent in the last weeks, days, and hours of life (Bruera, Franco, Maltoni, Wantanbe, & Suarez-Almazor, 1995; Kuebler, 1997).

Pathophysiology/Etiology

A direct relationship exists between underlying disease processes and agitated behaviors. Patients with dementia often will exhibit agitation. Alterations that occur within the brain contribute to changes in cognition, predominately in memory, judgment, and impulse control. Agitation can be a result of dementia, pain, depression, anxiety, constipation, or dyspnea (Bruera et al., 1995; Kuebler, English, & Heidrich, 2001). An agitated state also can be the result of drug intoxication or withdrawal (Bruera et al., 1995). Agitation contributes to a poor sense of well-being and quality of life (Kuebler et al.).

Manifestations

- Anxiety (most common manifestation)
- Hyperkinesia
- Aimless wandering
- Hyperactivity
- Pacing
- Hypervigilence

- Cursing
- Hypersensitivity (light/noise)
- Screaming, calling out, or arguing
- Verbal agitation or hiding, hoarding actions
  These manifestations can be either aggressive or nonaggressive.

Management

A. Death is not imminent.
   1. Initial onset of agitation usually presents rapidly, and treating the underlying cause is considered paramount.
   2. Neurocognitive alterations may be a result of opiate metabolites; therefore, either dose reduction or an alternate opiate should be considered (Bruera et al., 1995).
   3. Consider prolonged use of benzodiazepines as a contributing factor.
   4. If agitation persists, refer to the Delirium/Acute Confusion and Terminal Sedation sections.

B. Death is imminent.
   1. Symptomatic treatment of nonspecific agitation is appropriate at the end of life.
   2. Detection and correction of the underlying cause of agitation is considered the best intervention whenever possible.
   3. Early assessment and prompt intervention of agitation will decrease the onset of delirium.
      a) Hypodermoclysis ($)—can be used to reduce toxic medication metabolites contributing to agitation (Bruera et al., 1995).
      b) Haloperidol (Haldol®) ($)—titrating dose 0.5–2 mg po bid and prn q 4–6 hr
      c) Risperidone (Risperdal®) ($$), 3–6 mg po qd; olanzapine (Zyprexa®), 5–10 mg po qd; and quetiapine (Seroquel®), 150–750 mg po qd
   4. Maintain a soothing and comfortable environment that includes familiar surroundings, such as music and photographs (Allen, 1999).
   5. See Complementary Therapies.

Patient Outcomes

Agitation is resolved or minimized.

Professional Competencies

A. Identify early onset and recognition of the manifestations contributing to agitation.

B. Avoid the development and incidence of agitation with prompt assessment and intervention.

C. Rule out any reversible causes of agitation and treat appropriately.

D. Establish a soothing and comfortable environment.

E. Titrate medications to effect.

F. Keep medication metabolites to a minimum, and provide hydration, if needed.

References

Allen, L. (1999). Treating agitation without drugs. *American Journal of Nursing, 99*(4), 36–41.

Bruera, E., Franco, J., Maltoni, M., Wantanbe, S., & Suarez-Almazor, M. (1995). Changing patterns of agitated impaired mental status in patients with advanced cancer: Association with cognitive monitoring, hydration, and opioid rotation. *Journal of Pain and Symptom Management, 10,* 287–291.

Kuebler, K. (1997). *Hospice and palliative care clinical practice protocol: Terminal restlessness.* Pittsburgh: Hospice and Palliative Nurses Association.

Kuebler, K., English, N., & Heidrich, D. (2001). Delirium, confusion, agitation, and restlessness. In B. Ferrell & N. Coyle (Eds.), *Textbook of palliative nursing* (pp. 290–308). New York: Oxford University Press.

Kuebler, K., & Heidrich, D. (2001). Perspectives on end-of-life care. In J.M. Black, J.H. Hawks, & A. Keene (Eds.), *Medical surgical nursing: Clinical management for positive outcomes* (6th ed.) (pp. 447–460). Philadelphia: W.B. Saunders.

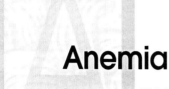

Anemia

Peg Esper, MSN, RN, CS, AOCN®

Definition

Anemia is a decrease in the circulating red blood cells, resulting from some underlying disorder. It may be seen as an acute or chronic condition.

Pathophysiology/Etiology

Patients with cancer or chronic illness often develop anemia. The cause is generally multifactorial and may include chemotherapy treatment, radiation therapy, nutritional deficits, blood loss, or damaged bone marrow (Griffin, 1998). The resulting overall effect of anemia can severely affect the patient's quality of life (Esper & Redman, 1999). Appropriate treatment of anemia as part of palliative care should be based on the uniqueness of each patient's situation.

Manifestations

- Fatigue
- Weakness
- Shortness of breath
- Malaise
- Dizziness/orthostasis
- Headache
- Cold intolerance
- Tachycardia/tachypnea
- Pallor

(Loney & Chernecky, 2000)

Management

A. Death is not imminent.
    1. Iron supplements ($)—Ferrous sulfate, 325 mg po tid. Beneficial if the individual is iron deficient (indicated by a decreased serum ferritin). Iron

supplements can have a number of unpleasant side effects, such as gastrointestinal upset and constipation. They are readily available and inexpensive to administer.

2. Blood transfusion ($$)—Administration early in care often can palliate symptoms but also may provide no benefit. Patient evaluation post-transfusion should occur to evaluate for a decrease in symptoms. In situations where bone marrow is compromised, blood transfusions serve a very temporary benefit, if any. Careful justification of transfusion should be made before initiating this treatment (Monti, Castellani, Berlusconi, & Cunietti, 1996).

3. Erythropoietin administration ($$$)—Use of erythropoietin agents is debatable in palliative care settings. Its use may decrease cancer-related fatigue, but it may not benefit all individuals. Weekly injections include side effects, such as fever, chills, and bone pain. Its benefit generally is not seen for several weeks following initiation of treatment and requires that patients have adequate ferritin levels for it to be effective. Concurrent administration of iron is recommended. Hematocrit levels should be checked regularly, and a dose reduction should be made if hematocrit is > 36% or an increase of > 4 points is seen in a two-week period (Micromedex, Inc., 2001). The cost of this agent may not be covered by the patient's insurance. Anticipated benefits should be evaluated carefully prior to use in this setting.

B. Death is imminent.
1. Attempts to treat manifestations of the anemia and not the anemia itself should be instituted.
2. Interventions include oxygen (nasal cannula, as masks often make people feel they are suffocating), rest, warm clothing, and blankets. Avoid sudden movements.

Patient Outcomes

A. Correction of anemia when feasible

B. Relief of anemia-associated symptoms

Professional Competencies

A. Manifestations of anemia are recognized early in the course of care.

B. The appropriateness of therapeutic versus palliative intervention is determined by individual patient evaluation.

C. Effectiveness of interventions is assessed regularly, and the treatment plan is modified, as necessary, for optimal patient outcomes.

Measurement Instruments

See the Fatigue and Dyspnea sections.

References

Esper, P., & Redman, B.G. (1999). Supportive care, pain management, and quality of life in advanced prostate cancer. *Urology Clinics of North America, 26,* 375–389.

Griffin, J.D. (1998). Hematopoietic growth factors. In V.T. DeVita, S. Hellman, & S.A. Rosenberg (Eds.), *Cancer: Principles and practice of oncology* (5th ed.) (pp. 2639–2652). Philadephia: Lippincott-Raven.

Loney, M., & Chernecky, C. (2000). Anemia. *Oncology Nursing Forum, 27,* 951–962.

Micromedex, Inc. (2001). *Healthcare series.* Greenwood Village, CO: Author.

Monti, M., Castellani, L., Berlusconi, A., & Cunietti, E. (1996). Use of red blood cell transfusion in terminally ill cancer patients admitted to a palliative care unit. *Journal of Pain and Symptom Management, 12,* 18–22.

Anorexia, Cachexia, and Nutritional Support

Suzanne W. Dixon, MPH, MS, RD, and Peg Esper, MSN, RN, CS, AOCN®

Definition

Anorexia is defined as a lack of appetite, whereas cachexia is the disordered metabolism characteristic of certain diseases or conditions, including, but not limited to, cancer, sepsis, chronic infections, HIV/AIDS, and other conditions resulting in systemic inflammation. Cachexia and subsequent anorexia can lead to weight loss, loss of muscle mass, loss of functional status, and decline in quality of life for patients with advanced illnesses.

Pathophysiology/Etiology

Anorexia is a lack of appetite resulting in an involuntary decline in food intake. Anorexia is an *effect* of cachexia rather than the *cause* of cachexia. Patients with cancer often develop cachexia. The cause is not completely understood but is thought to result from overproduction of proinflammatory (procachectic) mediators called cytokines and interferons. Tumor necrosis factor, interleukins 1 and 6 (IL-1 and IL-6), and interferon gamma (IFN-g) are believed to be among the more important mediators of the cachexia response (Barber, Ross, & Fearon, 2000; Marian, 1998; Tisdale, 2000a, 2000b).

The presence of these mediators can result in anorexia, hypermetabolism, and alterations in normal metabolic pathways. In simple starvation, the body readily adapts to calorie deficit by shifting to fatty acids as a major source of energy, thereby preserving lean body mass. In the cachectic state, the body fails to make this adaptation, which can lead to disproportionate wasting of lean body mass and loss of strength and functional status. This can result in a decline in the quality of life for the terminally ill patient (Barber et al., 2000; Cox & McCallum, 2000; Marian, 1998; Tisdale, 2000a, 2000b).

Manifestations

- Anorexia
- Weight loss

- Lean body mass loss
- Weakness
- Early satiety
- Malaise
- Anemia
- Dehydration
- Electrolyte imbalances
- Taste alterations
- Fatigue
- Lethargy
- Micronutrient deficiency

Management

A. Death is not imminent: Treat and manage symptoms that may affect nutritional intake and desire to eat, including constipation; bloating; diarrhea; feelings of fullness, early satiety, and poor appetite; altered sense of taste/smell; dry mouth or thick saliva; sore mouth/throat; nausea/vomiting; and pain.

   1. General measures (patient tips)

     a) Constipation (See Constipation.)

     b) Bloating (Cox & McCallum, 2000)

       (1) Limit beverages and foods that cause gas, such as carbonated drinks, broccoli, cabbage, cauliflower, cucumbers, peppers, beans, peas, onions, and garlic.

       (2) Lessen the amount of air swallowed by limiting talking while eating.

       (3) Avoid using straws to drink.

       (4) Avoid chewing gum.

     c) Diarrhea (See Diarrhea.)

     d) Feelings of fullness, early satiety, and poor appetite (Cox & McCallum, 2000)

       (1) Eat several meals and snacks each day instead of three larger meals.

       (2) Make eating more enjoyable by setting an attractive table, playing favorite music, or watching television.

       (3) Keep snacks handy to eat immediately (hunger may only last a few minutes), such as granola bars, nuts, pudding, chips, crackers, pretzels, trail mix, fruit, and one-serving sizes of tuna or chicken.

       (4) Eat favorite foods any time of day (e.g., if breakfast foods are appealing, eat them for dinner).

       (5) Eat every few hours—avoid waiting for hunger to occur.

       (6) Treat food like medicine—set times to eat, such as every 1–2 hours, and be sure to have at least 1–2 bites of some food at each "medication" time (quantity and type of food are less important; frequency of eating is more important).

   (7)   Eat small, frequent meals.
   (8)   Drink high-calorie, high-protein drinks, such as shakes and liquid supplements.
   (9)   Try fortified juice-based supplements such as Enlive!® (Ross, Abbott Park, IL) if taste fatigue of other supplements is a problem.
   (10) Drink fluids between meals rather than with meals (i.e., separate liquids from solids).
e) Altered sense of taste/smell (Cox & McCallum, 2000)
   (1)   Be fastidious with mouth care.
   (2)   Avoid food smells.
   (3)   Avoid meal preparation by the patient.
   (4)   Try foods that have minimal odors and short cooking time, such as scrambled eggs, French toast, pancakes, oatmeal, and Cream of Wheat® (Nabisco, Parsippany, NJ).
   (5)   Season foods with tart flavors such as lemon, citrus, and vinegar (as long as the patient does not have a sore mouth or throat).
   (6)   Flavor foods with basil, oregano, rosemary, tarragon, mustard, catsup, or mint.
   (7)   Marinate and cook meats in sweet fruit juices, dressings, or wine, such as sweet and sour pork, chicken with honey glaze, or beef with burgundy wine or Italian dressing.
   (8)   Rinse mouth with tea, ginger ale, salted water, or baking soda and water to clear taste buds before eating.
   (9)   Suck on lemon drops or mints, or chew gum (but not with a sore mouth or throat; avoid sugarless gums and candies if diarrhea is present).
f) Sore mouth/throat (Cox & McCallum, 2000)
   (1)   Be fastidious with mouth care.
   (2)   Eat soft, bland foods, such as creamed soups, cooked cereals, macaroni and cheese, yogurt, pudding, mashed potatoes, eggs, custards, casseroles, cheesecake, and milk shakes.
   (3)   Drink through a straw to bypass mouth sores.
   (4)   Eat high-protein, high-calorie foods to speed healing.
   (5)   Blend or moisten foods with gravy, butter, cream, or sauces.
   (6)   Soften foods such as bread by soaking them in milk.
   (7)   Stick to nonacidic juices such as apple juice; peach, pear, or apricot nectars; and grape juice (do not use grape juice if diarrhea is present).
   (8)   Avoid tart, acidic, or salty beverages and foods such as citrus, pickled items, and tomato-based foods.
   (9)   Avoid alcohol, caffeine, and tobacco.
g) Nausea/vomiting (Cox & McCallum, 2000)
   (1)   Treat as indicated with antiemetics or pro-motility drugs taken exactly as prescribed (preventing nausea/vomiting is easier than treating it).

    (2) Eat small frequent meals and snacks (sometimes nausea lessens if the stomach is not empty).

    (3) Eat bland foods, such as oatmeal and other cooked cereals, pasta, rice, and potatoes.

    (4) Try warm, salty foods and liquids, such as soups or broths.

    (5) Try dry foods, such as crackers, toast, dry cereal, or breadsticks, every 1–2 hours.

    (6) Avoid food smells.

    (7) Avoid meal preparation by the patient.

    (8) Try foods that have minimal odors and short cooking time, such as scrambled eggs.

    (9) Choose foods that do not have a strong odor, such as plain baked chicken or mashed potatoes.

  (10) Avoid eating in a room that is warm or stuffy.

  (11) Use mouth rinses before and after meals.

  (12) Sip warm ginger ale.

  (13) Sip ginger tea, chamomile tea, or peppermint tea (avoid peppermint if reflux is a problem).

  (14) Sit up to eat.

  (15) Do not lie down for at least one hour after eating.

  (16) Limit dairy products if they tend to cause gas and bloating.

  (17) Avoid overly sweet, fatty, fried, or rich foods such as desserts and French fries.

  h) Dry mouth or thick saliva (See Xerostomia.)

  i) Pain (See Pain.)

2. Enteral nutrition support ($$$) (National Comprehensive Cancer Network Nutrition Support Panel, 2001)

  a) Enteral nutrition support may be an option if

    (1) It can contribute to quality or length of life in a meaningful way.

    (2) The patient wants it.

    (3) The patient has a functioning gut.

    (4) It is not contraindicated by conditions such as intractable nausea and vomiting, obstruction, or gastroparesis (may be able to bypass these with a jejunal feeding tube instead of a gastric feeding tube).

  b) Indications

    (1) Patient meeting < 50% of required nutrient intake orally for 5–7 days or more

    (2) Inadequate oral intake for five or more days

    (3) Protein-energy malnutrition

    (4) Severe dysphagia

  c) Contraindications

    (1) Intestinal obstruction, ileus, or hypomotility of the intestine

    (2) Severe, intractable diarrhea that is unresponsive to treatment (treatment of underlying infection, diet modification, antidiarrheals)

   (3) High-output enterocutaneous fistulas
   (4) Acute pancreatitis
   (5) Prognosis does not warrant aggressive nutritional support; this is an individual decision that must be discussed with patient and family and treated on a case-by-case basis.
 d) Starting enteral feeding
   (1) Consult a registered dietitian to determine nutrient needs and to select a formula (e.g., high protein, fiber containing, elemental) and administration method (i.e., pump, gravity feeding, bolus feeding).
   (2) Troubleshoot (see Table 1).

Table 1. Troubleshooting for Simple Enteral Feeding Problems[a]

Problem	Possible Causes	Solutions
Feeding tube clog *Note:* DO NOT try to clear blockage by inserting an object into the tube as this could injure the stomach lining or damage the tube; DO NOT use cranberry juice, other juices, meat tenderizer, or carbonated beverages to unplug tube; acidic products cause the protein in TF formulas to coagulate and form clogs.	Inadequate flushing before or after administering feedings or medications; trying to put anything other than feeding formula or crushed, dissolved medications through the tube	Attempt to flush tube with a syringe filled with 30 cc warm water; if unsuccessful, fill syringe with water and move plunger back and forth several times until tube clears; avoid excessive force when trying to unclog tube; use a product designed to dissolve clogs, such as Viokase®; if unsuccessful, call your homecare nurse, doctor, or registered dietitian.
Leakage around the tube	Improper positioning; too-rapid feeding rate; blocked tube; tube out of position	Patient should sit at least 45 degrees upright during feeding and for at least one hour after feeding; slow feeding rate by 25%–50%; use instructions above to unblock tube; check for tube out of position by measuring length of tube or looking for mark on tube; if tube is longer than it should be or if the mark is farther out, contact doctor, as the tube may need to be replaced.
Diarrhea	Too-rapid feeding rate; using formula with too-high osmolality; not enough fiber in the formula; maldigestion/malabsorption	Decrease rate of feeding; switch to isotonic formula; change all or some of feeding formula to a fiber-containing formula; use an elemental formula or a formula that contains medium chain triglycerides as a fat source.

[a] Contact a registered dietitian or physician if these measures fail to correct the problem.

Note. Based on information from University of Michigan Health System Food and Nutrition Services, 1998.

(3) Address micronutrient deficiencies ($)—If death is not imminent, use of vitamin and mineral supplements, such as an iron supplement for iron-deficiency anemia (microcytic) or vitamin B_{12} and folic acid supplements for macrocytic/megaloblastic anemia, may be beneficial. However, the benefit of such supplementation must be weighed against the potential discomfort it can cause. It may be more beneficial to discontinue vitamin and mineral supplements that contribute to gastrointestinal distress, nausea, constipation, or diarrhea if they diminish quality of life to a significant degree (Cox & McCallum, 2000). This issue must be discussed with the patient, family, and caregivers. The costs and benefits of supplementation should be decided on a case-by-case basis.

3. Parenteral nutritional support ($$$$)
   a) Parenteral nutrition is almost never indicated in the patient who is terminally ill for the following reasons.
      (1) Adds very little in terms of quality and length of life
      (2) Risks (e.g., infection, hepatic and renal complications, fluid management problems) often outweigh the benefits.
      (3) Very expensive
      (4) Requires frequent blood work (no less than weekly) and intensive management
      (5) Can contribute to other problems and complications, such as ascites, edema, and hepatic and renal complications
   b) The most important issue is to help the family and patient understand the costs and benefits of total parenteral nutrition on a case-by-case basis.

4. Pharmacologic support: A number of agents have been used to promote appetite in the patient who is terminally ill.
   a) Hydrazine sulfate ($)—has not been shown to be of any benefit in several randomized trials (Watanabe & Bruera, 1996).
   b) Cyproheptadine hydrochloride (Periactin®) ($$)—has been shown to cause a slight increase in appetite/intake but failed to prevent persistent weight loss (Watanabe & Bruera).
   c) Cannabinoids—dronabinol (Marinol®) ($$$) 5–10 mg po twice a day—recent studies of patients with AIDS showed an increase in appetite, with a trend toward stable weight and decreased nausea (Watanabe & Bruera).
   d) Corticosteroids ($)—decreased nausea, an increased sense of well-being, and an increased appetite have been documented, though no persistent increase in weight has been seen. The beneficial effects appear to be time-limited and must be balanced against long-term side effects of administration, including Cushing's syndrome, proximal myopathy, immunosuppression, and exacerbation of delirium (Watanabe & Bruera).

    e) Megestrol acetate (Mcgace®) ($$), 800 mg/day po—a number of studies have shown beneficial effects on both appetite and weight gain. The greatest benefit was noted with the 800 mg/day dose. Possible side effects include edema, thrombosis, and vaginal bleeding (Tait, 1999; Watanabe & Bruera).

    f) Recombinant growth hormone ($$$$), 0.1 mg/kg/day—approved by the U.S. Food and Drug Administration for the treatment of AIDS-related wasting (Tait).

B. Death is imminent.

1. Decreased food and fluid intake appears to be a normal part of the "physiology" of dying.

2. In the last few weeks to days of life, a marked decline is seen in the functioning of the upper and lower gastrointestinal system, as well as a decrease in sensations of taste and smell.

3. Education of family members and caregivers at this stage is very important.

4. Facilitate understanding that the physical sensations of "starving" are not present. The patient feels little discomfort strictly from decreasing nutrition status. Hunger is nonexistent, and forcing the issue of food often is counterproductive. It can result in resentment and decreased quality of life.

5. Maintenance of strength and nutrition status at this time is unrealistic. Caregivers should be encouraged to show love and support in ways that do not involve preparation or provision of food.

6. Dehydration also may be normal during the end stage of the dying process. Often, the only discomfort associated with dehydration is a dry mouth, which can be alleviated with sips of water, ice chips, or moistened swabs (Cox & McCallum, 2000). (See Dehydration.)

7. Artificial hydration and nutritional support at this time can decrease quality of life simply by the nature of their invasiveness. Starting these measures when death is imminent generally is not advised.

8. If artificial hydration or nutritional support is already in place, decreasing the amount of the infusion to 500–600 cc/day may help to avoid discomfort from increased urinary output, gastrointestinal and pharyngeal secretions, and pulmonary edema. Stopping hydration altogether is an option, if desired by the patient and family (Cox & McCallum).

9. According to the American Medical Association's Code of Ethics, human dignity is the primary obligation if it conflicts with prolonging life. All competent patients have the right to accept or reject any or all forms of medical treatment. If an advance directive is in place, this should specify patient desires with regard to supportive interventions, including fluids and artificial nutrition, at the end of life (American Medical Association, 2001).

10. If the patient expresses a desire for voluntary cessation of eating and drinking, the following issues must be considered and addressed (Byock, 2000; Miller, Fins, & Snyder, 2000; Quill & Byock, 2000a, 2000b).

    a) Patient characteristics: Persistent, unrelenting, otherwise-unrelieved symptoms that are deemed unacceptable to patient and family, including pain, seizures, weakness, and extreme fatigue

    b) Patient informed consent

        (1) Patient must be fully competent.

        (2) Patient must be fully informed of all treatment and symptom management options.

        (3) Patient must be evaluated by a mental health professional to rule out treatable depression or other mental health conditions; a second opinion is strongly recommended.

        (4) A written informed consent must be in place.

    c) Terminal prognosis: Typically days to weeks (possibly months)

    d) Palliative care: Must be available, in place, and able to adequately relieve suffering

    e) Family participation: Clinicians should strongly encourage discussion; consensus should be reached, if possible, among the patient, immediate family members, and caregivers.

    f) Patient incompetence: Food and fluids (oral) must not be denied from incompetent patients who are willing and able to eat.

    g) Second opinions: Must be obtained from experts in underlying disease, mental health, pain management, and palliative care

11. If all of these issues are addressed and managed, voluntary refusal of food and fluids may be an appropriate option. Artificial nutrition and hydration are considered life-sustaining medical therapies similar to medications, surgery, dialysis, mechanical ventilation, or other medical interventions. Therefore, decisions regarding this issue should be handled using the same ethical and legal standards as other interventions. If the benefits of an intervention outweigh the costs, it is justified. If it is not beneficial or if the costs are higher than the benefits, it is not justified. Discontinuation of nutrition and hydration generally is *not* considered justified in the following situations (Byock, 2000; Miller et al., 2000; Quill & Byock, 2000a, 2000b).

    a) The patient will die of malnutrition before he or she would succumb to the disease process. An example includes a patient with severe dysphagia secondary to head and neck cancer, in which the primary diagnosis will not result in death before malnutrition.

    b) Untreated mental health issues are present, such as depression.

    c) The patient has a strong desire to "get affairs in order," such as writing a will or attending a specific family event.

    d) A new acute, but treatable, diagnosis arises.

Patient Outcomes

A. Malnutrition, dehydration, micronutrient deficiencies, weakness, wasting, and weight loss are corrected when feasible.

B. When maintenance of nutrition and hydration status is no longer a reasonable goal, comfort needs are met, such as providing ice chips for a dry mouth, even if adequate hydration is no longer a goal.

C. Patient maintains control over his or her intake.

Professional Competencies

A. Early recognition of the manifestations of cachexia/anorexia and dehydration

B. Institution of measures to increase appetite, intake, and calories as appropriate

C. Recognition of the costs and benefits of artificial nutrition versus the invasive nature of such interventions

D. Effectiveness of interventions regularly assessed and the treatment plan modified to optimize patient comfort and dignity

Measurement Instruments

A. Twenty-four hour food recall

B. Comprehensive diet history

C. Nutrition needs assessment (calorie and fluid needs for maintenance of nutrition and hydration status), Harris-Benedict equation, and the fluid needs formula

References

American Medical Association. (2001). *AMA policy.* Retrieved July 20, 2001 from the World Wide Web: http://www.ama-assn.org

Barber, M.D., Ross, J.A., & Fearon, K.C. (2000). Disordered metabolic response with cancer and its management. *World Journal of Surgery, 24,* 681–689.

Byock, I. (2000). Completing the continuum of care: Integrating life-prolongation and palliation. *CA: A Cancer Journal for Clinicians, 50,* 123–132.

Cox, A., & McCallum, P.D. (2000). Medical nutrition therapy in palliative care. In P.D. McCallum & C.G. Polisena (Eds.), *The clinical guide to oncology nutrition* (pp. 143–149). Chicago: American Dietetic Association.

Marian, M. (1998). Cancer cachexia: Prevalence, mechanisms, and interventions. *Support Line, 20*(2), 3–12.

Miller, F.G., Fins, J.J., & Snyder, L. (2000). Assisted suicide compared with refusal of treatment: A valid distinction? University of Pennsylvania Center for Bioethics Assisted Suicide Consensus Panel. *Annals of Internal Medicine, 132,* 470–475.

National Comprehensive Cancer Network Nutrition Support Panel. (2001). *Guidelines of enteral feeding support*. Rockledge, PA: Author.

Quill, T.E., & Byock, I.R. (2000a). Responding to intractable terminal suffering. *Annals of Internal Medicine, 133,* 562.

Quill, T.E., & Byock, I.R. (2000b). Responding to intractable terminal suffering: The role of terminal sedation and voluntary refusal of food and fluids. *Annals of Internal Medicine, 132,* 408–414.

Tait, N. (1999). Anorexia-cachexia syndrome. In C. Yarbro, M. Frogge, & M. Goodman (Eds.), *Cancer symptom management* (2nd ed.) (pp. 183–208). Boston: Jones and Bartlett.

Tisdale, M.J. (2000a). Metabolic abnormalities in cachexia and anorexia. *Nutrition, 16,* 1013–1014.

Tisdale, M.J. (2000b). Protein loss in cancer cachexia. *Science, 289,* 2293–2294.

University of Michigan Health System Food and Nutrition Services. (1998). *Home tube feeding manual* (2nd ed.). Ann Arbor, MI: The Regents of the University of Michigan.

Watanabe, S., & Bruera, E. (1996). Anorexia and cachexia, asthenia, and lethargy. *Hematology/Oncology Clinics of North America, 10,* 189–204.

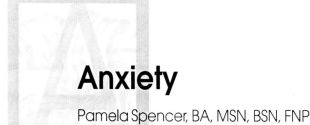

Anxiety

Pamela Spencer, BA, MSN, BSN, FNP

Definition

Anxiety may be described as fear of the unknown (not knowing what to expect) or fear of the known (knowing what to expect) (APA, 1994; Kuebler, English, & Heidrich, 2001). Anxiety is considered a universal experience. An anxious person experiences a vague, diffuse apprehension or uneasiness, often accompanied by feelings of uncertainty and helplessness (St. Marie, 2000). Anxiety is a subjective and observable experience. Its existence is either self-reported or inferred by observing behaviors. Anxiety is experienced along a continuum from mild to severe (St. Marie; Vachon, 1998). Mild anxiety may be beneficial because it serves as a motivator, whereas increased or sustained anxiety can be detrimental physiologically and psychologically (APA).

Pathophysiology/Etiology

Anxiety is triggered by the activation of the sympathetic nervous system, which involves the release of norepinephrine, creating a fight-or-flight response. Serotonin interacts with numerous receptor subtypes on different neurons, creating various psychobiologic functions that can be disruptive (Vachon, 1998). Anxiety is a symptom that has many causes, including physical, psychoemotional, and existential etiologies. Anxiety can occur in many different situations for patients living with advanced illness and should be regarded as a clinical spectrum ranging from normal to pathological (Vachon). Normal or reactive anxiety often is transient and is a direct response to stress or a perceived crisis. Adjustment disorder-reactive anxiety, on the other hand, is when the patient's anxiety exceeds 7–14 days (APA, 1994; Vachon). Organic anxiety often is the result of severe unrelieved symptoms (e.g., pain, dyspnea, unfinished emotional issues, side effects from medications, drug withdrawal) (Vachon). Cognitive changes or impairment can precipitate anxiety regardless of the underlying causes and can disrupt both the receiving and processing of sensory information (APA; Kuebler et al., 2001;

Vachon). This results in a diminished ability to handle stressful situations and creates the distressing sensation of anxiety.

Manifestations
Psychoemotional
- Tension
- Fears (nonspecific or specific)
- Difficulty concentrating
- Apprehension
- Irritability
- Nervousness

(APA, 1994; Kuebler, 2002)

Somatic
- Nausea
- Systolic hypertension
- Headache
- Chest pain/pressure
- Tachycardia/tachypnea
- Insomnia/restlessness
- Palpitations
- Dyspnea
- Tremors
- Weakness
- Sweating/flushing
- Diarrhea
- Dizziness
- Dilated pupils

(Kuebler, 2002; Kuebler et al., 2001; St. Marie, 2000; Vachon, 1998)

Management

A. General measures
  1. Anxiety-reducing techniques ($)—guided imagery, breathing exercises, music therapy, therapeutic touch, massage/Reiki, biofeedback, aromatherapy (See Complementary Therapies.)
  2. Psychotherapy ($$)—professional counseling individual/group
  3. Medication therapy ($–$$)
     a) Benzodiazepines
        (1) Lorazepam (Ativan®) ($) 0.5–1.0 mg/day po q 4–6 hours
        (2) Diazepam (Valium®) ($) 2–40 mg/day po q 4–6 hours
        (3) Clonazepam (Klonopin®) ($) 1–6 mg/day po q 4–6 hours
        (4) Chlorazepate (Tranxene®) ($) 7.5–90 mg/day po q 4–6 hours
        (5) Alprazolam (Xanax®) ($$) 0.75–4 mg/day po q 4–6 hours

     b) Phenothiazines: Chlorpromazine (Thorazine®) ($) 10–100 mg po titrated to effect q 4–6 hours

     c) Antianxiety agents: Buspirone (BuSpar®) ($$) 5 mg po tid, may increase in increments of 5 mg/day q 2–3 days to achieve optimum effect (daily dose not to exceed 60 mg)

     d) Antipsychotics: Haloperidol (Haldol®) ($) 0.5–2 mg po titrated to effect q 4–6 hours

  4. Oxygen ($$)

  5. Opiates ($–$$$) if related to pain or dyspnea

Patient Outcomes

A. Anxiety is resolved or maintained at a level where the ability to function is not impaired.

B. The impact anxiety has on perceived quality of life is articulated.

Professional Competencies

A. Identify anxiety that is disrupting the patient's ability to participate in desired activities.

B. Treat anxiety based upon severity of presentation.

C. Identify and treat potential medical conditions (e.g., fluid overload, electrolyte imbalances, endocrine and neurologic abnormalities, dyspnea, blood disorders/malignancies, medication side effects) contributing to anxiety.

D. Facilitate consultation with a psychologist or psychiatrist for patients experiencing debilitating anxiety levels.

E. Introduce pharmacologic interventions, in a timely fashion, with attention to pharmacokinetics.

References

American Psychiatric Association. (1994). *Diagnostic and statistical manual of mental disorders* (4th ed.). Washington, DC: Author.

Kuebler, K. (2002). Anxiety. In K. Kuebler, P. Berry, & D. Heidrich (Eds.), *End-of-life care: Clinical practice guidelines for advanced practice nursing* (pp. 199–212). Philadelphia: W.B. Saunders.

Kuebler, K., English, N., & Heidrich, D. (2001). Delirium, confusion, agitation and restlessness. In B. Ferrell & N. Coyle (Eds.), *The textbook of palliative nursing* (pp. 290–308). New York: Oxford University Press.

St. Marie, B. (2000). Anxiety. In D. Camp-Sorrell & R. Hawkins (Eds.), *Clinical manual for the oncology advanced practice nurse* (pp. 133–134). Pittsburgh: Oncology Nursing Press.

Vachon, M. (1998). The emotional problems of the patient. In D. Doyle, G. Hanks, & N. MacDonald (Eds.), *Oxford textbook of palliative medicine* (2nd ed.) (pp. 883–907). London: Oxford University Press.

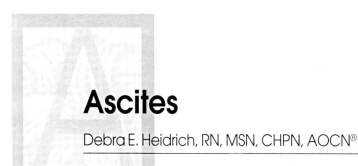

Ascites

Debra E. Heidrich, RN, MSN, CHPN, AOCN®

Definition

Ascites is an accumulation of excessive fluid in the peritoneal cavity.

Pathophysiology/Etiology

Ascites results from either a decrease in fluid being reabsorbed from the peritoneal cavity or an excessive production of peritoneal fluid. Constriction of the main thoracic duct or other lymphatic channels by tumor will impede the normal movement of fluid out of the peritoneal cavity. Peritoneal seeding with tumor leads to decreased capillary resistance and increased fluid accumulation. In patients with advanced liver disease, usually cirrhosis, a combination of sodium retention, portal hypertension, and decreased osmotic pressure causes excess fluid to leak into the peritoneal cavity. These factors also may contribute to the ascites associated with congestive heart failure and nephrotic syndrome (Bain, 1998; von Gunten & Twaddle, 1998; Walczak & Heckman, 1999).

Manifestations

- Dyspnea and orthopnea
- Weight gain
- Abdominal distention
- Abdominal pressure, discomfort, or pain
- Anorexia, early satiety, or indigestion
- Constipation
- Urinary frequency
- Edema of lower extremities
- Penile and scrotal edema
- Skin of abdomen taut and shiny

- Fatigue
- Tachycardia
- Nausea and vomiting
- Shifting dullness on percussion
- Fluid wave
- Diminished or high-pitched bowel sounds

(Heidrich, 2002; Twycross, 1997)

Management

A. General measures
  1. Elevate head of bed.
  2. Encourage small, frequent feedings and increase protein.
  3. Employ measures to prevent constipation/maintain bowel function.
  4. Encourage the patient to wear loose-fitting clothing.
  5. Elevate lower extremities when sitting.
  6. Encourage meticulous skin care.
  7. Give analgesics as needed.
  8. Place indwelling Foley catheter for urinary retention.

(Bain, 1998; Heidrich, 2002; Twycross, 1997)

B. Death is not imminent.
  1. Diuretic therapy ($–$$)—This intervention may be ineffective in malignant ascites and can deplete intravascular volume (Twycross, 1997; Waller & Caroline, 2000).
      a) Spironolactone (Aldactone®) 100–200 mg po/day is more effective than loop diuretics.
      b) If spironolactone is not effective alone, add a loop diuretic, such as furosemide (Lasix®) 40 mg po/day.
      c) Both medications can be increased to a maximum of 400–500 mg spironolactone and 160 mg furosemide.
      d) When satisfactory results are achieved, titrate to lowest effective dose, reducing loop diuretic first.
  2. Sodium and water restriction ($)—Restrict dietary intake of sodium to 2 g/day and water to 1.5 liters/day. Consider the benefit of this in relation to the impact on quality of life (Bain, 1998).
  3. Paracentesis ($$$)—May be performed to provide relief from symptoms.
      a) Monitor for hypotension when more than 1 liter of fluid is removed. Up to 5 liters may be removed safely from patients with malignant ascites (Bain; von Gunten & Twaddle, 1998).
      b) Consider infusion of albumin 40 g IV before and 6–8 hours after paracentesis when removing more than 2 liters of fluid from people with nonmalignant ascites (von Gunten & Twaddle).
      c) Monitor for catheter-related infection.
      d) Consider ostomy bag over puncture site for leakage of fluid.

(1) Pros
   (a) Removes large volume of fluid rapidly
   (b) Rapidly improves patient comfort
   (c) Simple procedure to perform in home or clinic
(2) Cons
   (a) Can lead to fluid/electrolyte imbalances
   (b) Fluid can reaccumulate in a matter of days.
   (c) Increased risk of infection seen with repeat procedures
   (d) Potential for bowel perforation
4. Peritoneovenous shunts ($$$$)—LeVeen™ catheters or Denver ascites shunts have one-way pressure-sensitive valves that allow shunting of fluid from the abdomen to the superior vena cava (Tueche & Pector, 2000).
5. Tenckhoff catheter ($$$)—Implanted catheter to provide steady removal of ascitic fluid (Lee, Lau, & Yeong, 2000)
6. Intraperitoneal therapy ($$$–$$$$)—Sclerosing by instillation of chemo-therapeutic agent
7. Octreotide (Sandostatin®) ($$$$)—Administration of 200–400 mcg sq/day has been reported to be effective in some cases of intractable ascites. The true cost-benefit ratio of this intervention has not been adequately evaluated (Cairns & Malone, 1999; Waller & Caroline, 2000).

C. Death is imminent.
   1. Position for comfort.
   2. Continue to remove abdominal fluid via paracentesis if this promotes comfort for patient.
      a) If a catheter has been placed for drainage of abdominal fluid, the cost and discomfort associated with the procedure is minimal and can greatly enhance comfort.
      b) If needle puncture is required, the discomfort associated with the procedure must be weighed against the potential increase in comfort. In addition, in the event arrangements cannot be made to perform this procedure at the patient's current location, the physical, emotional, and financial burdens of transporting the patient to a clinic or hospital must be evaluated.

Patient Outcomes

A. Relief of abdominal discomfort

B. Relief of dyspnea and orthopnea

C. Optimal control of ascites

D. Regular bowel movements

Professional Competencies

A. Recognize signs of increasing abdominal girth and discomfort.

B. Evaluate response to treatment, and modify the plan to prevent complications of therapies (e.g., overuse of diuretics, hypotension).

C. Use strict sterile technique for paracentesis.

D. Identify signs and symptoms of peritonitis promptly.

E. Instruct caregivers on the appropriate administration of medications, positioning techniques, care of paracentesis or peritoneal catheter site, and signs and symptoms to report to healthcare professionals.

Measurement Instruments

A. Abdominal girth measurements assist in evaluating effectiveness of interventions and changes in status over time. Measurements should be discontinued when death is imminent.

B. Dyspnea associated with ascites may be rated on a numeric scale to monitor effectiveness of interventions and changes in status over time.

C. Intake and output

D. Weights

References

Bain, V.G. (1998). Jaundice, ascites, and hepatic encephalopathy. In D. Doyle, G.W.C. Hanks, & N. MacDonald (Eds.), *Oxford textbook of palliative medicine* (2nd ed.) (pp. 557–571). New York: Oxford University Press.

Cairns, W., & Malone, R. (1999). Octreotide as an agent for the relief of malignant ascites in palliative care patients. *Palliative Medicine, 19,* 429–430.

Heidrich, D. (2002). Ascites. In K. Kuebler, P. Berry & D. Heidrich (Eds.) *End-of-life care: Clincial practice guidelines for advanced practice nursing* (pp. 189–198). Philadelphia: W.B. Saunders.

Lee, A., Lau, T.N., & Yeong, K.Y. (2000). Indwelling catheters for the management of malignant ascites. *Supportive Care in Cancer, 8,* 493–499.

Tueche, S.G., & Pector, J.C. (2000). Peritoneovenous shunt in malignant ascites. The Bordet Institute experience from 1975–1998. *Hepato-Gastroenterology, 47,* 1322–1324.

Twycross, R. (1997). *Symptom management in advanced cancer* (2nd ed.). Abingdon, England: Radcliffe Medical Press.

von Gunten, C.F., & Twaddle, M.L. (1998). Diagnosis and management of ascites. In A.M. Berger, R.K. Portenoy, & D.E. Weissman (Eds.), *Principles and practice of supportive oncology* (pp. 217–221). Philadelphia: Lippincott-Raven.

Walczak, J., & Heckman, C. (1999). Ascites. In C.H. Yarbro, M.H. Frogge, & M. Goodman (Eds.), *Cancer symptom management* (2nd ed.) (pp. 405–414). Boston: Jones and Bartlett.

Waller, A., & Caroline, N.L. (2000). *Handbook of palliative care in cancer* (2nd ed.). Boston: Butterworth-Heinemann.

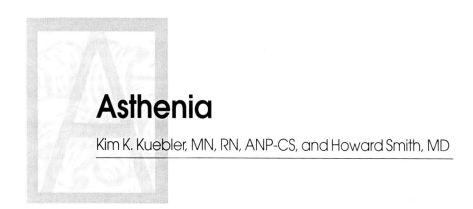

Asthenia

Kim K. Kuebler, MN, RN, ANP-CS, and Howard Smith, MD

Definition

Asthenia is generalized physical weakness, with an absence or loss of strength. It can be multifactorial and includes both physical and mental fatigue (Bruera & Fainsinger, 1998; Bruera & MacDonald, 1988; Lichter, 1990).

Pathophysiology/Etiology

Asthenia commonly is encountered at the end of life and accompanies various etiologies (e.g., infection, dehydration) and metabolic disturbances (e.g., hypercalcemia, hypokalemia, hypothyroidism, hypoadrenalism). Other factors may include anemia, insomnia, depression, prolonged immobility, and medications (e.g., phenothiazines, antidepressants). Additionally, paraneoplastic syndromes (e.g., Eaton-Lambert syndrome), myelopathy, myopathies, and neuropathies also may be responsible. The progression of terminal disease (e.g., malignancies, tumor burden) and other chronic medical conditions can lead to asthenic symptoms (Bruera & Fainsinger, 1998; Bruera & MacDonald, 1988; Lichter, 1990).

Manifestations

- Anxiety
- Cachexia
- Agitation
- Insomnia
- Fatigue
- Weakness
- Depression
- Lethargy
- Anorexia

(Bruera & Fainsinger, 1998; Bruera & MacDonald, 1988; Lichter, 1990)

Management

A. General measures (Bruera & Fainsinger, 1998; Bruera & MacDonald, 1988)
1. The clinician should attempt to find out exactly what the patient means by weakness—is the weakness a result of physical or mental fatigue?
2. Does the patient experience generalized weakness or is the patient's perception that of having a low energy level?
3. Does the patient associate this weakness with worsening disease or impending death? Is the weakness acute or slowly progressive?

B. Death is not imminent (Bruera & Fainsinger, 1998; Bruera & MacDonald, 1988; Lichter, 1990).
1. The treatment of asthenia should focus on assessing and managing specific manifestations or identifying reversible causes.
2. Pharmacologic management of asthenia
    a) Prednisone ($)—5–30 mg po qd
    b) Cylert (Pemoline®) ($$)—18.75–75 mg po qd (chewable)
    c) Methylphenidate (Ritalin®) ($$)—5–10 mg po bid
    d) Dextroamphetamine (Dexedrine®) ($$)—2.5 mg po bid
    e) Megestrol acetate (Megace®) ($$$)—800 mg po qd may improve some asthenic symptoms.
3. Transfuse blood products ($$)—as appropriate
4. Erythropoietin ($$$)—therapy as needed

C. Death is imminent.
1. Provide education and support to patient and family.
2. Encourage the establishment of realistic goals, and identify patient priorities.
3. Promote balance between rest and activities as well as conservation of energy to "gear up" for important events (e.g., daughter's wedding).

Patient Outcomes

A. Maintain or regain physical/mental strength.

B. Maintain optimal sense of well-being.

C. Complete unfinished business.

D. Conserve energy for important events.

Professional Competencies

A. Identify and evaluate reversible causes of or factors contributing to asthenia.

B. Help patient to set realistic goals based upon current condition.

C. Arrange realistic therapy based upon the patient's goals and the extent of illness.

D. Use pharmacologic interventions to optimize the patient's performance status.

References

Bruera, E., & Fainsinger, R. (1998). Clinical management of cachexia and anorexia. In D. Doyle, G. Hanks, & N. MacDonald (Eds.), *Oxford textbook of palliative medicine* (2nd ed.) (pp. 548–557). New York: Oxford University Press.

Bruera, E., & MacDonald, N. (1988). Asthenia in patients with advanced cancer. *Journal of Pain and Symptom Management, 3,* 9–14.

Lichter, I. (1990). Weakness in terminal illness. *Palliative Medicine, 4*(2), 73.

Bereavement

Jerre Cory, MA, CSW, and Kim K. Kuebler, MN, RN, ANP-CS

Definition

Bereavement refers to the experience of having suffered a loss (Campbell, Geller, Smellie-Decker, & Kuebler, 2000). It is interesting to note that the words *bereave* and *rob* derive from the same root, which implies an unwilling deprivation by force, having something withheld unjustly and injuriously, a stealing away of something valuable.

Specific Issues Related to Palliative Care
Individual Variation and Duration Patterns

Probably the most frequently asked question about grief and bereavement concerns duration. Bereavement is extremely individual and includes a myriad set of factors that may influence the duration of bereavement. Individual factors include the following:

Psychologic factors: These include but are not limited to the nature of loss—was it sudden, planned, or anticipated? What was the relationship with the deceased? Was it an emotionally close relationship or estranged and difficult? Is the deceased the wage earner, the problem solver, the one who made all of the decisions? Was the deceased the social motivator in a group, labeled the life of the party? Were there important emotional issues that were never discussed or were left unfinished? Are there issues that the bereaved needs to reconcile?

Individual coping skills: Is the mourner able to problem-solve alone, or has he or she always relied on the deceased? Individuals' past experiences with death and dying invade current bereavement. The influences of culture, age, ethnicity, education, social supports, and religion directly affect grief and bereavement. Additional stressors, such as illness or other losses, will influence the ability to cope.

Physiologic factors: Poor nutrition and lack of sleep and exercise can exacerbate an already-difficult life experience. Substance use often is increased when difficult issues, such as loss, are encountered. Prolonged substance abuse precludes the acceptance of loss and can impede the bereavement process (Parkes, 1998).

Strategies to Promote Optimal Bereavement

A. Perform ongoing evaluation and assessment of the bereaved; this is important after the death experience. Grief is considered the beginning phase of bereavement (Rando, 1997). Identification of complicated grief at the onset offers a better prognosis. Uncomplicated reactions of acute grief may last several months and, in some specific cases, even longer. In contrast, uncomplicated mourning can last for a number of years, if not a lifetime in some circumstances. Many clinicians can assist the bereaved in the acute process by allowing them to express their reactions to the loss; this should be performed with an emphasis on reorienting in relation to the deceased, the self, and the external world (Parkes, 1998).

B. Acknowledge that the expression of bereavement is an individual response. Individual dynamics are as unique as the patients themselves. The myriad variables that determine the bereavement process as described above ultimately will influence the ability to move on. The first year of bereavement usually is associated with greater morbidity and mortality (Campbell et al., 2000).

C. Initiate community referrals for supportive services. The Medicare hospice benefit provides for bereavement services as well as those available through funeral homes and local clergy.

Outcomes

A. Bereaved individuals receive appropriate referral and resources to promote a healthy bereavement process.

B. Bereaved individuals have the opportunity to tell their stories of the dying/death experience.

C. Bereavement occurs within the individual's personal time frame.

Professional Competencies

A. Incorporate knowledge of community resources to assist the bereaved in a supportive and therapeutic way.

B. Transfer the relationship to another professional or other caring individuals (e.g., therapist, support-group system, friends of the mourner).

C. Provide reassurance to the bereaved that mourning is a normal process.

References

Campbell, M., Geller, S., Smellie-Decker, M., & Kuebler, K. (2000). Grief: Strategies for people anticipating or recovering from a loss. *Michigan Nurse, 73*(5), 14–23.

Parkes, C. (1998). Grief. In D. Doyle, G.W.C. Hanks, & N. MacDonald (Eds.), *Oxford textbook of palliative medicine* (2nd ed.) (pp. 995–1010). New York: Oxford University Press.

Rando, T. (1997). *Treatment of complicated mourning.* Champaign, IL: Research Press.

Bowel Obstruction

Pamela Spencer, BA, MSN, BSN, FNP

Definition

Bowel obstruction is caused by an occlusion of the lumen of the intestine or lack of normal propulsion, which prevents or delays intestinal content from passing along the gastrointestinal tract (Baines, Oliver, & Carter, 1985). Obstruction may be the presenting symptom of cancer or may develop during the course of malignancy (Woodruff, 1997). Any site in the bowel can be affected, from the gastroduodenal junction to the rectum and anus.

Pathophysiology/Etiology

Partial or complete obstruction often is multifactorial. Mechanical etiologies include luminal obstruction from cancer, constipation, or obstipation (fecal impaction). Pseudo-obstruction can occur from obstipation or paralytic ileus. Wall infiltration or stricture formation can result from cancer, radiation, surgery, or benign peptic ulcer disease (Baines et al., 1985). Sources of extrinsic compression include cancer or adhesions (surgical or malignant). Paralytic obstruction can result from disruption of autonomic nerve supplies from retroperitoneal infiltration or spinal disease. Other causes may include medications (e.g., opiates, anticholinergics), postoperative surgical complications, peritonitis, metabolic involvement from hypokalemia or hypercalcemia, radiation fibrosis, or arterial/venous insufficiency (Baines et al., 1985; Brennis, Perry, Read-Paul, & Bruera, 1998; Woodruff, 1997).

Manifestations

- Nausea/vomiting (occurs in 100% of patients with complete obstruction)
- Emesis (Early onset in small-bowel obstruction, especially following oral intake. Feces may have originated from large-bowel obstruction.)
- Abdominal/visceral pain (colicky or cramping pain near the site of obstruction)

- Changes in bowel sounds (Complete obstruction causes an absence of bowel sounds; partial obstruction results in high-pitched sounds or tympany.)
- Tympanic sounds with percussion of abdomen (especially if distended)
- History of infrequent bowel movements (constipation)
- Absence of flatus (with complete obstruction)

(Baines et al., 1985; Brennis, Perry, Read-Paul, & Bruera, 1998; Woodruff, 1997)

Management

A. Death is not imminent.
1. Nasogastric intubation and fluid replacement can be used temporarily ($$).
2. Pharmaceuticals
    a) Antiemetics ($) (Brennis et al., 1998; Skidmore-Roth, 1999; Woodruff, 1997)
        (1) Prochlorperazine (Compazine®) 5–10 mg po q 6–8 hours
        (2) Metoclopramide (Reglan®) 10 mg po q 4–6 hours or 40–60 mg over a 24-hour sq infusion
    b) Analgesics ($–$$$)—Opiate therapy as needed for relief of pain
    c) Anticholinergics ($)—Scopolamine hydrobromide 0.4 mg sq q 4–6 hours or 0.6–1.2 mg over a 24-hour sq infusion
    d) Somatostatin analog ($$$$)—Octreotide (Sandostatin®) 0.1 mg sq or 0.2–0.3 mg over a 24-hour sq infusion
    e) Corticosteroids ($)—Dexamethasone (Decadron®) 8–16 mg po/sq
3. Surgical interventions ($$–$$$$) should be considered in acute or complete obstruction, peritonitis, strangulated hernia, or gastric outlet obstruction.

B. Death is imminent (Brennis et al., 1998; Skidmore-Roth, 1999; Woodruff, 1997).
1. Manual removal of fecal impaction ($), various enemas
2. Pharmaceutical management
    a) Stool softener ($)—Docusate sodium (Colace®)
    a) Dexamethasone (Decadron®) ($)—20 mg sq bid for 24 hours then taper to lowest effective dose for reduction of symptoms
    c) Hyoscyamine butylbromide (Levsin®) ($)—10–20 mg sq q 4 hours (q 1 hour prn)
    d) Octreotide (Sandostatin®) ($$$$)—50–100 mcg sq bid
3. Insert nasogastric tube for decompression and pain control.
4. Provide appropriate mouth care.

Patient Outcomes

A. Optimal comfort is maintained.

B. Obstruction is reversed whenever possible.

C. Maintain regular bowel movement.

Professional Competencies

A. Evaluate and appropriately identify underlying causes of obstruction.

B. Initiate therapy based upon the extent of illness and the patient's and family's goals of care.

C. Provide patient and family education.

References

Baines, M., Oliver, D., & Carter, R. (1985). Medical management of intestinal obstruction in patients with advanced malignant disease: A clinical and pathological study. *Lancet, 2,* 990–903.

Brennis, C., Perry, B., Read-Paul, L. & Bruera, E. (1998). *Ninety-nine questions and answers about palliative care: A nurses' handbook.* Edmonton, Canada: Regional Palliative Care Program.

Skidmore-Roth, L. (1999). *Mosby's 1999 nursing drug reference.* St. Louis, MO: Mosby.

Woodruff, R. (1997). Bowel obstruction. In R. Woodruff (Ed.), *Symptom control in advanced cancer* (pp. 28–30). Melbourne, Australia: Asperula Publisher.

Caregiver Burden

Jerre Cory, MA, CSW, and Kim K. Kuebler, MN, RN, ANP-CS

Definition

The term *caregiver* can be applied to anyone who provides assistance to someone who is in need. Formal caregivers refer to paid professional providers or trained volunteers. Informal caregivers include members of the patient's family or his or her friends. *Caregiver burden* describes the multiple demands that are placed upon informal caregivers when caring for their loved one (Ferrell, Grant, Borneman, Juarez, & Ter Veer, 1995).

Specific Issues Related to Palliative Care

A. Informal caregivers, usually 65 years of age or older, provide the majority of care in the United States (Derby & O'Mahony, 2001).
  1. Spouses account for the majority of caregivers, with the female being the primary caretaker (Ferrell et al., 1995).
  2. Unpaid care giving is provided for an estimated 1–4 years, and more than 20% of caregivers provide direct care for their loved ones for more than five years (Schott-Baer, Fisher, & Gregory, 1995).
  3. Men are more likely to be cared for by their wives, and women receive care predominately from children or children-in-law.

B. Americans are living longer, increasing the demands on informal caregivers. People who are living longer with advanced illness may be pushing the capacities of familial caregivers to the limit. Most of these patients experience functional limitations that cause them to require daily assistance when performing routine activities.

C. Financial concerns exacerbate caregiver burden.
  1. The elderly often are not aware of community-based services that can help them to meet their in-home physical care needs.
  2. Families with low socioeconomic status, low literacy levels, and minimal support systems are at greater risk of caregiver burden (Weitzner, McMillan, & Jacobson, 1999).

D. Informal caregivers often are reluctant to seek additional support.
　　1. Physical care demands upon the caregiver may become problematic as the patient's disease progresses.
　　2. A bed-bound patient who requires repositioning and wound care and has incontinence issues may become overwhelming for the caregiver who is reluctant to seek assistance or facilitate support from other family members.
　　3. The demands of constant care that accompany changes in cognition affect caregiver coping.

Strategies to Decrease Caregiver Burden

A. Perform ongoing assessment and evaluation of the patient's and caregiver's needs.
　　1. Most elderly patients living with advanced illness prefer to remain home during the last years of life.
　　2. The elderly often will require varying levels of assistance with personal care needs, meal preparation, maintenance of healthcare appointments, errands, and various social commitments.
　　3. As illness progresses, so do the patient's physical care needs.
　　4. Caregivers who are elderly may not be aware of what the physical, emotional, and social demands entail when choosing to care for their loved ones at home.

B. Empower patients to remain at home, with an emphasis on care for the caregiver.

C. Evaluate realistic expectations by both the patient and his or her caregiver(s).
　　1. Assessment includes an understanding of the disease process and the complications associated with disease progression.
　　2. Financial resources determine where to focus referrals (i.e., Medicaid Waiver Program versus private-pay providers).
　　3. Reassure patients and their caregivers that efforts to help the patient remain at home will be a priority.

Community Resources

A. Hospice
　　1. If the patient has a prognosis of less than six months to live, he or she is eligible for hospice services, which provide numerous caregiver support services, including respite care (Weitzner et al., 1999).
　　2. If the patient is having prolonged unmanaged symptoms, he or she qualifies for continuous nursing care (in home) under the Medicare hospice benefit (Derby & O'Mahony, 2001).

B. Medicaid Waiver Program

1. Considered a "nursing home without walls"; however, not all states participate in this program, and very few will support Medicaid hospice services along with the Medicaid Waiver Program (Kuebler & Moore, in press).
2. This program offers comprehensive formal care giving in the home to people with limited financial resources.

C. Senior services: Most communities have senior service resources that provide home health aides, meals-on-wheels, transportation, and access to other valuable resources.

D. Senior day care: A European model that provides respite for caregivers; this may be available in some communities.

Caregiver Outcomes

A. Maintains optimal well-being and is able to accomplish self-goals

B. Recognizes physical, emotional, and social limitations resulting from caregiving demands

C. Establishes a trusting relationship with professional supports and participates in the patient's plan of care

D. Utilizes community resources based upon individual needs

Professional Competencies

A. Evaluate the effectiveness of outside resources, and modify the plan of care accordingly with caregiver participation.

B. Identify changes in the patient's care demands and seek timely interventions.

C. Be familiar with community-based resources.

References

Derby, S., & O'Mahony, S. (2001). Elderly patients. In B.R. Ferrell & N. Coyle (Eds.), *Textbook of palliative nursing* (pp. 435–449). New York: Oxford University Press.

Ferrell, B., Grant, M., Borneman, T., Juarez, G., & Ter Veer, A. (1995). Family care giving in cancer pain management. *Journal of Palliative Medicine, 2,* 185–195.

Kuebler, K. & Moore, C. (in press). *The Michigan advanced practice palliative care self-training manual.* Lansing, MI: Michigan Department of Community Health.

Schott-Baer, D., Fisher, L., & Gregory, C. (1995). Dependent care, caregiver burden, hardiness, and self-care agency of caregivers. *Cancer Nursing, 18,* 299–305.

Weitzner, M., McMillan, S., & Jacobson, P. (1999). Family caregiver quality of life: Differences between curative and palliative cancer treatment settings. *Journal of Pain and Symptom Management, 17,* 418–428.

Communication
Karen J. Stanley, RN, MSN, AOCN®, FAAN

Definition

Living with advanced illness that is no longer responsive to traditional biomedicine intensifies the importance and value of therapeutic communication. Therapeutic communication between patients and their family members, caregivers, and friends provides an open, nonjudgmental venue to explore thoughts, feelings, and expressions of meaning. Conversations that are patient-focused and driven can lend powerful intervention to many nonresponsive symptoms. Positive, healthy communication also can influence the coping, grieving, and bereavement of the patient's loved ones (Larson & Tobin, 2000).

Specific Issues Related to Palliative Care: Barriers to Effective Communication

A. Clinicians vary widely in their ability to elicit relevant information from their patients (Kristjanson, 2000).
   1. A patient often will disclose significantly more information surrounding his or her emotional and social functioning when the healthcare provider has a positive attitude toward the psychosocial care aspects of the patient and his or her family.
   2. Therapeutic communication is inhibited by using closed-ended questions.
   3. Discomfort with death and dying issues will impede therapeutic communication.

B. Patient and family reluctance
   1. Denial, anger, fear, and generalized anxiety often can distract the patient and his or her family from articulating issues that they find important.

C. Death denying/defying culture
1. The cultural phobias surrounding death and dying in the United States are problematic when encouraging therapeutic conversations.
2. The discomfort associated with discussions of death and dying interferes with the clinician's skills and may conflict with values that are traditional in the biomedical setting.
3. Death often is viewed as failure, and discussions often surround aggressive interventions versus palliative care options.

Strategies to Maintain Optimal Communication

A. Identify barriers to effective therapeutic communication: Recognize that patient denial, anger, fear, generalized anxiety, or social withdrawal can negatively affect communicating with the patient about his or her important issues.

B. Encourage discussions of advance directives and future care planning.
1. Query the patient's feelings and values concerning his or her illness.
2. Investigate the patient's concerns, related to unfinished business.

C. Providing the therapeutic use of self
1. Therapeutic communication can only occur when listening skills that encourage patients to tell their stories are practiced (Stanley, 2000).
2. Therapeutic use of self provides a mutual participatory relationship that is not dominated by controlling the conversation.
3. By using less directive skills such as silence, paraphrases, reflections, and sincerity, the clinician is able to provide structure to the conversation yet empower the patient to express his or her needs.
4. Offering self promotes opportunities for discussion and demonstrates a willingness to hear painful fears and worries that family members may have difficulty dealing with emotionally.

D. Provide difficult information in a culturally appropriate manner.
1. Most patients and families have a need for as well as a right to information concerning:
   a) Prognosis
   b) Pathophysiologic sequelae (i.e., expected symptomatology) of the illness
   c) Plan of care for expected symptomatology
   d) Potential side effects of palliative care interventions
   e) Plan of care for side-effect management
2. This information can reduce the fear of the unknown and ease the psychologic process of dying.
   a) If the patient/family needs help in asking questions of other healthcare providers, assist them to prepare a list of appropriate questions.

      b) It is imperative to determine what kind of and how much information a patient and family wish to have and who is to hear it.

E. Encourage communication between the patient and his or her family.
  1. Help to identify barriers that lead to family and friends refusing to discuss the realities of illness, particularly if the patient wishes to have these specific conversations.
  2. Patients who are not given the opportunity to communicate important issues may demonstrate self-isolation and can experience greater fear, anxiety, or depression.
  3. Family conferences may be appropriate to explore areas that patients report that they have been discouraged from discussing pertaining to their illness.

F. Appreciate the individuality of each patient's communication expressions.
  1. The varied approaches of communicating one's feelings may entail communicating through gestures, body language, facial expressions, and eye contact.
  2. 80% of communication is nonverbal, so understanding this form of communication is critical.

G. Explore the patient and family's perception of realistic expectations.
  1. Therapeutic communication that is focused on reasonable goals of care will determine the patient's understanding of his or her prognosis (Garg, Buckman, & Kason, 1997).
  2. Gradual and gentle conversations can help transition patients and their families to acknowledge the irreversible nature of their illness.

Patient Outcomes

A. Participates in active and open communication concerning important issues and needs

B. Experiences meaningful relationships with people who are important to them

C. Resolves personal issues surrounding unfinished business

Professional Competencies

A. Recognize communication barriers and help facilitate patient-centered discussions.

B. Offer the therapeutic use of self through listening and a nonjudgmental appreciation of the patient and his or her family.

C. Evaluate what the patient and family know about the illness and prognosis.

D. Do not assume that everyone *should* accept his or her terminal prognosis. Meet people where they are, and help to gently move them toward healthy discussions on issues of importance.

E. Use and encourage a collaborative interdisciplinary approach of care.

References

Garg, A., Buckman, R., & Kason, R. (1997). Teaching medical students how to break bad news. *Canadian Medical Association Journal, 156,* 1159–1164.

Kristjanson, L.J. (2000). Establishing goals: Communication traps and treatment lane changes. In B.R. Ferrell & N. Coyle (Eds.), *Textbook of palliative nursing* (pp. 331–338). New York: Oxford University Press.

Larson, D., & Tobin, D. (2000). End-of-life conversations evolving practice and theory. *JAMA, 284,* 1573–1578.

Stanley, K.J. (2000). Silence is not golden: Conversations with the dying. *Clinical Journal of Oncology Nursing, 4,* 34–40.

Complementary Therapies

Nancy K. English, PhD, APN, CS

Definition

Complementary therapies (CTs) are nonpharmacologic interventions designed to complement, enhance, and support the patient's quality of life. The clinician can use modalities such as massage, music, and aromatherapy as a means of providing another method of therapeutic support to patients and their families.

Specific Issues Related to Palliative Care

An increasing number of adults in the United States have used some form of CT to manage chronic pain, anxiety, and fatigue—symptoms commonly encountered in palliative care (Astin, 1998). The increasing interest in and use of CTs has led to the development of the Center for Complementary and Alternative Medicine within the National Institutes of Health (NIH). NIH and others recognize that CT interventions have a positive outcome when used in combination with traditional interventions (Spencer & Jacobs, 1999).

Evaluating the Appropriateness of Complementary Therapy

The following concerns should be addressed:
- Patient and family familiarity, comfort level, and interest in the use of CT
- Patient and family expectations regarding the outcomes of CT
- Expertise and credentials of the individual offering or teaching the family CT
- Experience of the CT practitioner with patients and families within the palliative care setting

- Evidence-based research or empirical studies supporting the use of CT
- Legal or ethical implications of specific interventions
- Cost of education, time, and materials needed for implementation of specific interventions

Methods of Complementary Therapy

A. Aromatherapy
1. Definition: Aromatherapy is the use of fragrances and essences from plants to affect or alter a person's mood or behavior and to facilitate physical, mental, and emotional well-being. The chemicals composing essential oils in plants have a host of therapeutic properties and have been used historically in Africa, Asia, and India (Stevenson, 1998).
2. Essential oils (see Table 1)

Table 1. Essential Oils and Their Indications

Essential Oil	Indications
Lavender (*Lavandula angustifolia*)	Insomnia, anxiety, agitation (Cavanagh & Wilkinson, 2000; Kyle, 2000)
Bergamot (*Citrus bergamia*)	Depression and grief (Davis, 1995)
Cypress (*Cupressus sempervirens*)	Transition (death imminent), breathing difficulties (Kerr, 2000)
Spikenard (*Nardostachys jatamansi*)	Anxiety, fear at time of death (Davis, 1991)

3. Death is not imminent.
    a) Hydrotherapy baths: Mix 8 drops essential oil with ½ oz. mild liquid soap; add to bath.
       (1) Allow patient to stay in bath at least 10 minutes.
       (2) Teach the patient to focus inward on breathing, inhaling and exhaling in a slow and rhythmic pattern.
    b) Massage
       (1) Add 18 drops essential oil to 30 ml grape-seed oil or the cream or lotion preferred by patient/family.
       (2) Precautions for topical applications of oils
          (a) Do not use with patient who is undergoing chemotherapy. Wait seven days following chemotherapy infusions (Casey, 2000).
          (b) Only use pharmacology-grade oils, as these are the most pure.
          (c) Do not massage or use oils when patient is febrile.
          (d) Use light massage only when platelet count is low (Casey).

        (e) Prior to beginning a massage, ask the patient to focus for a few moments on his or her breathing, gradually slowing the breathing.

    c) Diffuser (minute molecules of oil are diffused in the air)
        (1) Add 10–12 drops oil to designated port.
        (2) Place in patient's room for 20–30 minutes.

    d) Compress
        (1) Place 5–10 moist washcloths in an electric "hot pot" on low.
        (2) Add 5 drops essential oil.
        (3) Warm for 10 minutes.
        (4) Offer compress to patient after morning care or at bedtime and prn (Kyle, 2000).

    e) Candles: Aromatherapy candles, with scents of choice, can be purchased at specialized candle stores.

    f) Atomizer or spritzer
        (1) Add 15 drops essential oil to 3 oz. (90 ml) distilled water or purified water in an atomizer.
        (2) Spray the atomizer. (Lavender or cypress may be helpful for the patient experiencing breathlessness, as they help reduce associated anxiety.)

  4. Death is imminent: Anointing
    a) Place 2 or 3 drops oil on a cotton ball or tissue, and lightly touch the cotton ball to the forehead of the patient.
    b) Spiritual caregivers or family can offer prayer, poetry, song, or family ritual.

B. Therapeutic touch
  1. Definition: Therapeutic touch (TT) is a consciously directed process of energy exchange through the practitioner's hands to balance the recipient's energy field. This practice is derived from "laying on of hands" as practiced by many indigenous cultures and religions (Ash, 1997; Macrae, 1994).
  2. TT assumes that health equals a balance in the individual's energy field.
  3. Disease is represented by disruptions and imbalances in the energy field.
    a) An individual experiences an energy field imbalance with a variety of symptoms, such as anxiety, depression, pain, or muscle tension.
    b) TT attempts to restore balance and thus offer relief of symptoms (Macrae, 1994).
    c) TT's potential in the palliative care setting is for symptom relief as well as spiritual care.
  4. TT is performed by individuals trained in the specifics of this technique (see Resources).

C. Reiki
  1. Definition: Reiki (pronounced "ray-kee") is a gentle, hands-on healing art. A Reiki intervention consists of a series of approximately 12 hand posi-

tions. The Reiki practitioner's hands are placed on the patient in a pre-scribed order.

2. A Japanese scholar and educator, Mikao Usui, instituted the Usui System of Reiki healing during the early 20th century in Japan, where Reiki is widely practiced today. Hawayo Takata, a Japanese American woman, brought it to the United States in 1937 (Haberly, 2000).

3. This noninvasive complementary intervention is easily learned and can help patients achieve a relaxed and calm state of mind.

4. It may be used as a stand-alone intervention, in conjunction with massage, or with other holistic interventions.

5. The practitioner needs to complete approximately 10 hours of level 1 Reiki training in the Usui System of Reiki healing. A master teacher in the Usui System offers specific treatment patterns and guidelines for the Reiki session.

D. Music therapy
1. Definition: The therapeutic use of music in the palliative care setting has been widely documented as a beneficial complementary intervention in pain and symptom relief (Burns, Harbuz, Hucklebridge, & Bunt, 2001; Petterson, 2001; Rykov & Salmon, 1998). The psychologic (mind-body) effect of music on individuals depends on the intent of the clinician's goal for the intervention. The clinician may use music as an adjunct along with other CTs (e.g., music with massage) or as a source of distraction during painful or stressful medical/nursing interventions (Broscious, 1999; Chlan, 1998).

2. Emphasis
   a) Select music according to the desired intent and outcomes.
      (1) The patient's preferences for prescriptive music must be considered first and foremost.
      (2) The order of the movement (rhythm) of the music is the second key component. The correct rhythm can synchronize the rhythm of the patient's heart and respiratory rate (Chlan & Tracy, 1999).
   b) The melody of a selected piece accounts for the emotional or psychologic response.
      (1) The melody becomes symbolic for communication with buried memories.
      (2) These memories often are tucked away in the unconscious realms of the mind, thus creating emotional responses to the music (e.g., it feels good, sad, happy; it does nothing) (Chlan & Tracy).
   c) Specific rhythms, along with melody, can be used to evoke the underlying emotion.
      (1) Usually the emotional response is individual, whereas the clinician can adjust rhythm to obtain a desired physiologic response, such as relaxation. The patient's preference may be Big Band music or rap. The rhythm selected can be 4/4, a slow rap, or a

waltz, if the prescriptive therapeutic effect is relaxation or distraction.

(2) The body rhythm and a pleasant memory (body-mind) are in harmony with the music, creating a sense of calm, albeit momentarily, for the patient.

(3) The "chalice of response," a melodious harp, is played in many inpatient/palliative care settings when death is imminent (Horrigan, 2001).

5. Interventions

  a) Adjunctive—played in conjunction with allopathic or complementary interventions

   (1) Selection of music without words—sounds of nature such as birds, the ocean, classical pieces, or New Age harmonics

   (2) Distracting—relaxation is desired when adverse or painful stimulus is anticipated or current.

   (3) Interview patient/family as to favorite music or music that holds special memories or meaning.

   (4) Instruct family or primary caregiver when to play specific music (e.g., during traumatic or invasive procedures).

   (5) During life-review sessions—remembering happy, sad, or joyful times

  b) Transcending—death is imminent.

   (1) Select music that is slow and mellow.

   (2) Discuss choices with family if patient is unable to make a selection as to what he or she would prefer.

   (3) Create a sacred space (i.e., in the home setting, scented candles and lowered lights may be appropriate).

E. Additional useful complementary therapies in palliative care (The following require specialized education and supervised practice.)

  1. Acupuncture—Traditional practice of Chinese and Korean medicine where needles are placed in designated areas on the body according to where energy blockages are diagnosed. This form of treatment is made in a variety of ways, most often by pulse diagnosis, which reveals energy imbalance within the body. NIH is in consensus that acupuncture is an effective intervention in a variety of conditions (Bareta, 1998; Villaire, 1998). The credentialing organization is the Accreditation Commission of Acupuncture and Oriental Medicine, and the resulting license is Licensed Acupuncturist (Leake & Broderick, 1999).

  2. Art therapy—Art therapy offers the opportunity for a creative expression whereby the patient can explore fears and emotions that may not surface in talking therapies. It can uncover unconscious strengths within the mind that aid the patient in finding hope in seemingly hopeless circumstances. Requirements for practice include a postdegree education and an internship with a practicing therapist (Pratt & Wood, 1997).

Patient Outcomes

A. Increased sense of relaxation
1. Decrease in muscle tension, especially in facial expression (relaxed eyes)
2. Unlabored respiration
3. Calm voice
4. Statements of patient or caregiver that reflect relaxation

B. Decreased sense of suffering and abandonment perceived when facing death

C. Verbal or nonverbal expression of safety and trust in caregivers

D. Increased sense of well-being perceived by patients (Quality-of-life measurements reveal an increased sense of control regarding matters of daily living and death.)

Professional Competencies

A. Identify the goal of CT with the patient or family.

B. Provide information on CT to patient/family as nonpharmacologic interventions.

C. Use good judgment when selecting CTs in the clinical setting or referring to a complementary therapist.

D. Provide instruction to patient and family when feasible on specific types of CT.

E. Evaluate and document the patient's response to CT.

Resources

A. American Music Therapy Association: www.musictherapy.org

B. Healing Touch International: www.healingtouch.net

C. Kyle, Laraine, MSN, RN, classes for healthcare professionals: www.aroma-rn.org; larainek@qwest.net (e-mail)

D. National Association of Aromatherapy: www.NAHA.org

E. Nurse-Healers Professional Associates: www.therapeutic-touch.org

F. Reiki teachers: www.musictherapy.org; dssbuckley@aol.com (e-mail)

References

Ash, C.R. (1997). Therapeutic touch: Healing through the hands. *Complementary Medicine for the Physician, 2*(1), 1, 6–8.

Astin, J.A. (1998). Why patients use alternative medicine: Results of a national study. *JAMA, 279,* 1548–1553.

Bareta, J. (1998). Evidence presented to consensus panel on acupuncture's efficacy. *Alternative Therapies in Health and Medicine, 4*(1), 22–29.

Broscious, S.K. (1999). Music: An intervention for pain during chest tube removal after open heart surgery. *American Journal of Critical Care, 8,* 410–415.

Burns, S.J., Harbuz, M.S., Hucklebridge, F., & Bunt, L. (2001). A pilot study into the therapeutic effects of music therapy at a cancer help center. *Alternative Therapies in Health and Medicine, 7*(1), 48–56.

Casey, M. (2000, February). Aromatherapy in the care of cancer patients and their families. *Aromatherapy Today,* pp. 10–14.

Cavanagh, H.M., & Wilkinson, J. (2000, September). Lavender: The essential oil? *Aromatherapy Today,* pp. 40–42.

Chlan, L. (1998). Effectiveness of a music therapy intervention on relaxation and anxiety for patients receiving ventilatory assistance. *Heart and Lung, 27,* 169–176.

Chlan, L., & Tracy, M.F. (1999). Music therapy in critical care: Indications and guidelines for intervention. *Critical Care Nursing, 19*(3), 35–41.

Davis, P. (1991). *Subtle aromatherapy.* Essex, England: C.W. Daniel.

Davis, P. (1995). *An A–Z aromatherapy.* New York: Barnes & Noble Press.

Haberly, H.J. (2000). *Reiki, Hawoyo Takata's story* (9th ed.). Olney, MD: Archedigm Publications.

Horrigan, B. (2001). Therese Schroeder-Sheker: Music thanatology and spiritual care for the dying. *Alternative Therapies in Health and Medicine, 7*(1), 69–77.

Kerr, J. (2000, June). Essential oil profile—Cypress. *Aromatherapy Today,* pp. 8–10.

Kyle, L. (2000, November). *End-of-life care with aromatherapy.* Proceedings at the Pacific Institute of Aromatherapy Conference, San Francisco, CA.

Leake, R., & Broderick, J. (1999). Current licensure for acupuncture in the United States. *Alternative Therapies, 5*(4), 94–96.

Macrae, J. (1994). *Therapeutic touch: A practical guide.* New York: Alfred A. Knopf.

Petterson, M. (2001). Music for healing: The creative arts program at the Ireland Cancer Center. *Alternative Therapies in Health and Medicine, 7*(1), 88–89.

Pratt, M., & Wood, M. (1997). *Art therapy creative expression in palliative care.* London: Routledge.

Rykov, M., & Salmon, D. (1998). Bibliography for music therapy in palliative care, 1963–1997. *American Journal of Hospice and Palliative Care, 15,* 174–180.

Spencer, J.W., & Jacobs, J.J. (1999). Complementary/alternative medicine: An evidence-based approach. St. Louis, MO: Mosby.

Stevenson, C. (1998). Aromatherapy. In D. Rankin-Box (Ed.), *The nurses' handbook of complementary therapies* (pp. 51–58). London: Churchill-Livingstone.

Villaire, M. (1998). NIH consensus conference confirms acupuncture's efficacy. *Alternative Therapies, 4*(1), 21–30.

Constipation

Kimberly A. Zielke, MD

Definition

Constipation is the passage of small, hard feces infrequently and with difficulty. Objective indicators include failure to defecate at least three times a week, straining with stools during more than 25% of defecations, and defecation lasting for more than 10 minutes (Sykes, 1998).

Pathophysiology/Etiology

A large number of patients with advanced illness develop constipation. Contributing factors include medications (opiates, anticholinergics, phenothiazines, antacids, diuretics, anticonvulsants, iron, antihypertensive agents), immobility, hypercalcemia, dehydration, inadequate food intake, low-fiber diet, confusion, direct effects of malignancy (obstruction, nerve damage), or concurrent disease (diabetes, hypothyroidism, hypokalemia, diverticular disease, hemorrhoids, colitis) (Sykes, 1998).

Manifestations

- Abdominal bloating
- Cramping, pain
- Loss of appetite
- Early satiety
- Confusion
- Diarrhea
- Rectal pain
- Hemorrhoids
- Small stool size
- Hard stool
- Straining to move bowels

- Urinary incontinence

(Caraccia-Economou, 2001; Curtis, 1999)

Management

A. Death is not imminent.
  1. Several prophylactic measures should be employed when possible. These include maintaining general symptom control, encouraging activity, maintaining adequate oral intake, anticipating the constipating effects of drugs (altering treatment or starting a laxative prophylactically), and creating a favorable environment (privacy, sitting upright) (Caraccia-Economou, 2001).
  2. A combination stimulant and softener is the most effective way to reduce constipation. This medication should be given around the clock to avoid a cyclic trend of constipation alternating with loose bowel movements. Start with a low dose and titrate upward. If loose bowel movements occur, hold for 24 hours and restart dose at one level down (Sykes, 1998).
      a) Casanthrol and docusate sodium (Peri-Colace®) ($)—1–2 tablets po bid no ceiling effect, also available in syrup
      b) Senna (Senokot®) ($)—1–3 tablets po bid or qid, may titrate both senna and docusate sodium until bowel movement occurs
      c) Senna concentrate and docusate sodium (Senokot S®) ($$)—same dosing as above for senna.
  3. When the amount of combination stimulant and softener medications produces distressing side effects (e.g., cramping), an osmotic agent should be added, such as the following (starting dose for all: 15 cc po bid).
      a) Milk of magnesia ($)
      b) Sorbitol ($)
      c) Lactulose (Chronulac®) ($$)
  4. Suppositories (glycerin, bisacodyl) or enemas (saline, oil retention, milk and molasses) ($)—can be considered when the patient requires assistance with evacuation. Suppositories may be adequate if only moderate softening is required. In patients whose rectal vault is loaded with soft stool, a suppository may assist in initial defecation, thus relieving some rectal discomfort. Manual disimpaction may be necessary to relieve discomfort.

B. Death is imminent.
  1. Even when a patient has had minimal intake for days or weeks, the bowels still need to move to provide comfort. Stool is not only a formation of food but also includes metabolic wastes. A patient who is dying may experience dysphagia, so a suppository or enema may be more useful than oral medication.
  2. If the patient is experiencing increased confusion, abdominal bloating, cramping or pain, then the following interventions should be considered. It is important to keep the rectal vault clear of stool when wanting to use the rectum for medication administration and bioavailability.

    a) Bisacodyl suppository (Dulcolax®) ($)
    b) Saline enema (Fleet®) ($)

Patient Outcomes

A. Soft bowel movements at regular intervals

B. Abdominal comfort, control, and reduction of accompanying symptoms (e.g., nausea, vomiting, confusion)

C. An empty rectal vault for administration of rectal medications

Professional Competencies

A. Recognize the need for bowel support in the majority of patients with advanced illness.

B. Incorporate stimulant/softeners for all patients receiving opiate medications.

C. Monitor bowel-movement patterns and institute interventions when no bowel movement occurs in three days.

D. Recognize that the symptoms of agitation, confusion, restlessness, abdominal bloating, nausea, and pain also can be indicators of constipation.

References

Caraccia-Economou, D. (2001). Bowel management: Constipation, diarrhea, obstruction, and ascities. In B. Ferrell & N. Coyle (Eds.), *Textbook of palliative nursing* (pp. 139–155). New York: Oxford University Press.

Curtis, C. (1999). Constipation. In C.H. Yarbro, M.H. Frogge, & M. Goodman (Eds.), *Cancer symptom management* (2nd ed.) (pp. 508–521). Boston: Jones and Bartlett.

Sykes, N. (1998). Constipation and diarrhea. In D. Doyle, G.W.C. Hanks, & N. MacDonald (Eds.), *Oxford textbook of palliative medicine* (2nd ed.) (pp. 513–521). New York: Oxford University Press.

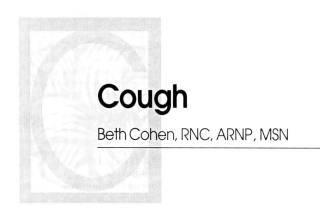

Cough

Beth Cohen, RNC, ARNP, MSN

Definition

Cough is an explosive expulsion of air from the lungs that acts as a protective mechanism to clear air passages or a symptom of pulmonary disturbance.

Pathophysiology/Etiology

Patients with chronic illness often develop a cough, usually related to pneumonia, congestive heart failure, and congestion because of an inability to clear their airway as a result of weakness or fatigue (Ahmedzai, 1998). Cough affects the patient's life by decreasing the ability to hold a conversation comfortably, inducing shortness of breath, gagging, vomiting, or scratchy throat. Ineffective cough allows for continuing congestion and a feeling of drowning in their own secretions. Cough may be dry and hacking or sputum producing.

Manifestations

- Shortness of breath
- Fatigue
- Weakness
- Tachycardia
- Chest pain
- Sore throat
- Wheezing
- Hemoptysis
- Gagging/vomiting

(Ahmedzai, 1998; Regnard & Tempest, 1998)

Management

A. General measures
  1. Treat underlying cause when possible.

2. Administer antibiotics if infection (e.g., bronchitis) is suspected.
3. Provide optimal hydration (Greif & Golden, 1994).
4. Provide optimal mobility (Greif & Golden).
5. Eliminate exposure to respiratory irritants (e.g., cigarette smoke, hair spray, dust, cleaning agents, body powder, perfumes) (Greif & Golden).

B. Death is not imminent.
1. Cough medications
   a) Several types contain narcotics, such as codeine, and help suppress a cough (antitussives), whereas others help patients bring up secretions (expectorants).
   b) Generally, side effects include gastrointestinal upset and diarrhea.
   c) Cough medications are available over the counter and by prescription and are generally inexpensive and administered orally in either liquid or gel tablet form.
   d) They are best used on a schedule rather than prn. Taste of the liquid form varies greatly.
   e) For coughs that do not respond to general cough suppressants, methadone syrup ($$) (5–10 mg po bid) sometimes is used for its long-lasting benefits (Greif & Golden, 1994; Hodgson & Kizior, 2001).
2. Humidification of the air/oxygen ($–$$)—This includes the use of a cool-mist vaporizer or humidifier in the home setting or a humidified oxygen source if the patient is on oxygen. The purchase of a humidifier/vaporizer is relatively inexpensive, and quiet ones are available in most drugstores. In a home setting, if the patient is strong enough, he or she can be helped to the bathroom and can inhale the steam from a hot shower. Be sure to guard against chill when leaving the bathroom. If on oxygen via nasal cannula, assess the nares frequently (Greif & Golden).
3. Suctioning—Remove secretions if cough is ineffective.
4. Benzonatate (Tessalon Perles®) ($$) 100 mg po tid (Hodgson & Kizior)
5. Nebulized xylocaine (Lidocaine®) ($) 5 ml 2% solution over 20 minutes or nebulized bupivicaine (Marcaine®) ($$) 5 ml 0.25% solution (may inhibit gag reflex) (Hodgson & Kizior)

C. Death is imminent.
1. All attempts to treat the cough noninvasively should be taken, with the focus on the patient's wishes and comfort.
2. Treatments may include oxygen via nasal cannula, rest, humidification, decreased stimulation, and decreased conversation with the patient, unless he or she wishes otherwise.

Patient Outcomes

A. Relief from cough and associated symptoms is achieved.

B. Adequate air exchange is maintained.

C. Comfort is maintained.

D. Cough does not interfere with patient's rest.

Professional Competencies

A. Underlying etiology of cough is identified early in the course of care when possible.

B. Interventions to control cough are determined and implemented.

C. Effectiveness of interventions is assessed regularly, and the treatment plan is modified as needed for optimal patient outcomes.

References

Ahmedzai, S. (1998). Palliation of respiratory symptoms. In D. Doyle, G.W.C. Hanks, & N. MacDonald (Eds.), *Oxford textbook of palliative medicine* (2nd ed.) (pp. 603–604). New York: Oxford University Press.

Greif, J., & Golden, B.A. (1994). *AIDS care at home.* New York: John Wiley & Sons.

Hodgson, B., & Kizior, R. (2001). *Saunders nursing drug handbook 2001.* Philadelphia: W.B. Saunders.

Regnard, C., & Tempest, S. (1998). *A guide to symptom relief in advanced disease.* Hale, England: Hochland & Hochland.

Cultural Awareness

Rev. James M. Deshotels, SJ, APRN

Definition

Cultural awareness is the ability to respect, understand, and enter into another person's culture. Establishing a cultural awareness allows successful interaction to occur at a meaningful human level to establish a therapeutic relationship. Cultural awareness does not mean achieving agreement or homogeneity with another but rather achieving a relationship of intersubjectivity and respect (Amenta, 1997; Eck, 1993; Mitty, 2001).

Specific Issues Related to Palliative Care

A. Return to cultural norms at the end of life: Patients and their families may return to cultural norms, thought patterns, and customs long hidden or ignored (Frankl, 1984; Mitty, 2001).

B. Cultural dissonance
    1. It can impede communication and compromise care, comfort, and the ability to process unfinished business.
    2. Cultural dissonance may result in isolation from family and significant others and require considerable patience.
    3. It may impede the effort to reconcile, put affairs in order, or express love.
    4. It also may alter perceptions of pain and comfort, impede communication with caregivers, and interfere with the achievement of therapeutic goals, especially if these are not mutually agreed upon.
    5. Cultural dissonance may interfere with the effort to identify and address social and economic needs (Singer, Martin, & Kelner, 1999; Stiles, 1990).

C. Patients outside mainstream culture
    1. These individuals may experience a sharper power gradient in the therapeutic relationship.

2. One of the challenges for healthcare providers is to understand that the scientific culture, though dominant, is not the only one, nor is it inherently superior or obvious to members of other cultures (Eck, 1993; Frankl, 1984; Institute of Medicine, 1997; Mitty, 2001; Singer et al., 1999; Stiles, 1990).

Strategies to Maintain Optimal Cultural Awareness

A. Educate interdisciplinary caregivers.
   1. Assessment, recognition, and acknowledgment of the existence of cultural diversity can facilitate communication among the patient, significant others, and the palliative care team.
   2. Ignorance of the patient's cultural norms and support systems can lead to cultural mistakes that are crisis provoking.

B. Mediate between the patient and family: The palliative care team can help address and activate the dominant culture in an attempt to help preserve the autonomy and comfort level of the patient and his or her family during a time of great stress.

C. Cultural awareness lies with the provider.
   1. The cultural power gradient associated with most therapeutic relationships in health care is coupled with the tendency for subcultures to be marginalized.
   2. It is extremely important for the provider to understand and respect the patient's culture rather than the other way around.

D. Facilitate cultural resources.
   1. The patient's capacity for intercultural dialogue may be compromised at the end of life.
   2. Accessing community resources is important for culturally diverse patients and families.

E. Clinical cultural competence (Fitzgerald, 1989; Institute of Medicine, 1997; Mitty, 2001; Reimer, Davies, & Martens, 1991; Stiles, 1990)
   1. Healthcare providers should develop an attitude of respect and willingness to learn from the patient and family about their cultural systems.
   2. Avoid imposing or assuming personal norms on members of other cultures.

Patient Outcomes

A. Optimal communication, respect, and dignity are achieved despite cultural diversity.

B. Cultural practices perceived as significant are followed and integrated into the plan of care (Institute of Medicine, 1997; Singer et al., 1999).

Professional Competencies

A. Acknowledge and become familiar with the various cultures and subcultures within one's practicing community.

B. Evaluate individual patient/family cultural preferences.

C. Demonstrate the ability to respect, understand, and enter into another person's culture.

D. Identify cultural resources to use within the local community.

E. Provide cultural interventions that will optimize quality of care.
(Institute of Medicine, 1997; Mitty, 2001; Reimer et al., 1991; Singer et al., 1999; Stiles, 1990)

References

Amenta, M. (1997). Guest editorial. Spiritual care: The heart of palliative nursing [Guest editorial]. *International Journal of Palliative Nursing, 3,* 1.

Eck, D. (1993). Challenge of pluralism. *Nieman Reports, 47,* 2.

Fitzgerald, F. (1989). Improve your skills in physical diagnosis: Learning to emulate Sherlock Holmes . . . extraeorporeal diagnosis. *Consultant, 29*(4), 63–74.

Frankl, V. (1984). *Man's search for meaning: An introduction to logotherapy* (3rd ed.). New York: Simon & Schuster.

Institute of Medicine. (1997). *Approaching death: Improving care at the end of life.* Washington, DC: National Academy Press.

Mitty, E. (2001). Ethnicity and end-of-life decision-making: Removing cultural blinders. *Reflections on Nursing Leadership, 27*(1), 28–31.

Reimer, J.C., Davies, B., & Martens, N. (1991). Palliative care: The nurse's role in helping families through the transition of "fading away." *Cancer Nursing, 14,* 321–327.

Singer, P.A., Martin, D.K., & Kelner, M. (1999). Quality end-of-life care: Patients' perspectives. *JAMA, 281,* 163–168.

Stiles, M. (1990). The shining stranger: Nurse-family spiritual relationship. *Cancer Nursing, 13,* 235–245.

Death and Dying

Debra E. Heidrich, RN, MSN, CHPN, AOCN®

Definition

Death is physiologically defined as the absence of a heartbeat and respirations. It is the expected outcome in the palliative care setting. Dying is a process that begins at birth. In the palliative care setting, the term *dying* most often refers to the final weeks, days, or hours of life.

Pathophysiology/Etiology

Many different pathophysiologic processes can lead to organ failure and eventual cessation of cardiac and respiratory function. These processes can include direct insult to the organ from the terminal disease (e.g., respiratory failure with lung cancer) or indirect insult to a vital system because of complications of the disease (e.g., heart block because of hypercalcemia). When one body system fails, others also are compromised and eventually fail. As this is often a slowly progressive process in the palliative care setting, signs and symptoms of body system failure may start subtly and become more profound as death approaches.

Manifestations

Symptoms the patient has been experiencing may become worse or subside as the disease progresses, and new symptoms may appear (Twycross & Lichter, 1998). Frequent assessment of the patient is required to identify troublesome symptoms early and intervene to promote comfort. General symptoms associated with the dying process include (Kemp, 1999; Storey, 1998; Twycross & Lichter)
- Muscle weakness
- Dysphagia
- Lethargy/drowsiness

- Decreased urinary output
- Skin discoloration
- Mottled skin
- Incontinence/retention
- Immobility
- Dyspnea
- Death rattle (noisy respirations)
- Cheyne-Stokes respiration
- Withdrawal from activities and relationships
- Decreased intake (natural dehydration of dying)
- Pale or bluish nailbeds, cool extremities.

"Nearing death awareness" (Callahan & Kelley, 1992) is a special knowledge of what dying and death is like and also of what the individual needs to die peacefully. Common themes of these experiences include
- Describing a place
- Talking to, or being in the presence of, someone who is not alive
- Knowledge of when death will occur
- Choosing a time of death
- Needing reconciliation
- Preparing for travel or change
- Being held back
- Symbolic dreams.

Confusion, agitation, and restlessness also may occur during the dying process (Twycross & Lichter, 1998).

Management

A. Death is anticipated in days.
1. Treat all symptoms aggressively with the goal of comfort. (See appropriate sections for the specific symptoms.) In most circumstances, treatment of pain should not be discontinued or decreased simply because that person can no longer report pain or can no longer swallow. This will precipitate an uncomfortable withdrawal.
2. Teach the family the signs and symptoms of dying, both to prepare them for the changes they will see and to assist them in recognizing when death is approaching.
3. Provide emotional and spiritual support for the patient and family, using an interdisciplinary approach.
4. Anticipate patient needs and evaluate for any potential discomforts that the patient may not be able to communicate clearly. The profound weakness associated with the dying process can lead to anxiety and fear. Educate the family regarding these changes.
5. Evaluate medication requirements and discontinue those that are no longer needed for medical management.

a) When the patient is not able to swallow medications, determine the best option for an alternate route of administration based on the patient's location (home versus inpatient facility), preferences, burdens associated with the alternate route, and available support systems.

b) The gastrointestinal tract is considered the least invasive and expensive route of medication administration.

    (1) Consult a pharmacist regarding which medications can be crushed, dissolved in water, or administered sublingually or buccally when swallowing is difficult.

    (2) Suppositories also are an option of this less expensive route, but around-the-clock rectal administration of medications may be objectionable to the patient and family. Consult a knowledgeable pharmacist to determine the need to increase, decrease, or maintain the oral dose when switching to the rectal route.

    (3) Some medications are available commercially in suppository form. Many medications made for oral administration can be administered rectally for symptom management by placing the pills in a gelatin capsule.

    (4) Subcutaneous or IV routes of administration also may be considered when the gastrointestinal tract is not an option.

6. Keep the patient's mouth clean and moist.
7. Monitor for urinary incontinence and intervene to keep skin clean and dry.
   a) Catheterization may not be required as output decreases.
   b) If turning and cleaning is uncomfortable for the dying patient or overly burdensome for the caregivers, catheterization is appropriate for the incontinent patient.
8. Monitor for urinary retention. Foley catheterization often is more comfortable than intermittent catheterization.
9. Treat the discomfort and anxiety associated with dyspnea. (See Dyspnea.)
10. Prepare the patient and family for nearing-death-awareness experiences. Some patients are reluctant to share these experiences for fear of being labeled crazy or confused. However, these experiences often are a source of comfort for both the patient and the family.
11. Treat confusion, agitation, and restlessness appropriately. (See individual sections.)

B. Death is anticipated in hours.
1. Continue to treat physical symptoms to achieve comfort.
2. Continue to evaluate the need for medications and discontinue as many as appropriate to maintain good symptom management. Be sure to consider the potential of withdrawal symptoms.
3. Teach family that skin mottling, peripheral hypoxia with pale or bluish nailbeds, and cool extremities are anticipated. The patient may or may not experience feeling cold. Blankets provide sufficient comfort. Heating devices (heating pads, hot-water bottles, packs heated in a microwave) should

be used with caution, if at all, as the patient may not be able to perceive or articulate if the device is too hot, causing tissue damage.

4. Decrease the distress associated with noisy respirations. Death rattle is probably more distressing to the family than to the patient. However, hearing is believed to remain intact longer than other senses, making this distressing to the patient, as well.

   a) Position changes may minimize noisy respirations. Positioning patients on their sides often prevents secretions from pooling at the top of the airway.

   b) Occasionally, suctioning the upper airway can remove pooled secretion. Avoid deep suctioning; it is painful and counterproductive, and stimulates more secretions.

   c) Anticholinergic medications dry secretions and can quiet noisy breathing (Storey, 1998; Twycross & Lichter, 1998). These agents are used with caution, as they can cause confusion and agitation. Meticulous mouth care will be required to treat the dry-mouth side effect. No studies are available comparing the benefits and burdens of the various anticholinergic agents used for this purpose.

      (1) Atropine 1% ophthalmic solution ($) 1–2 gtt sl bid–tid

      (2) Atropine ($+) 0.4–0.6 mg sq q 4 hours

      (3) Scopolamine transdermal patch (Transderm-Scop®) ($$)

      (4) Hyoscyamine (Levsin®) ($) 0.125–0.25 mg sl tid

      (5) Glycopyrrolate (Robinul®) ($) 1–2 mg po q 8 hours

5. Provide emotional and spiritual support for patient and family, using the interdisciplinary team.

Patient Outcomes

A. Optimal control of all symptoms to the time of death

B. Attainment of a peaceful death

Professional Competencies

A. Recognize signs and symptoms of approaching death.

B. Provide ongoing evaluation of interventions used to control symptoms to determine their appropriateness in the final days and hours of life.

C. Provide appropriate education to patients and caregivers regarding the dying process.

D. Provide patients and caregivers with emotional and spiritual support to promote healthy grieving.

References

Callahan, M., & Kelley, P. (1992). *Final gifts: Understanding the special awareness, needs, and communications of the dying.* New York: Bantam Books.

Kemp, C. (1999). *Terminal illness: A guide to nursing care* (2nd ed.). Philadelphia: Lippincott-Raven.

Storey, P. (1998). Symptom control in dying. In A.M. Berger, R.K. Portenoy, & D.E. Weissman (Eds.), *Principles and practice of supportive oncology* (pp. 741–748). Philadelphia: Lippincott-Raven.

Twycross, R., & Lichter, I. (1998). The terminal phase. In D. Doyle, G.W.C. Hanks, & N. MacDonald (Eds.), *Oxford textbook of palliative medicine* (2nd ed.) (pp. 977–992). New York: Oxford University Press.

Dehydration

Kim K. Kuebler, MN, RN, ANP-CS

Definition

Dehydration is an overall reduction of the body's total water content. This may be associated with the normal dying process when patients experience a lack of interest in food and water. Hyponatremic dehydration occurs when both salt and water are limited, and the body's electrolytes are in less proportion than water content (Ellershaw, Sutcliffe, & Saunders, 1995).

Pathophysiology/Etiology

Dehydration directly affects the body's blood volume and circulatory reserve. The lack of circulatory volume influences the body's baroreceptors. Dehydration is multifactorial and, if left untreated, can lead to multiorgan failure (Ellershaw et al., 1995).

Manifestations

- Opiate toxicities
- Hallucinations
- Confusion
- Hyperalgesia
- Restlessness
- Dry mucus membranes
- Myoclonus
- Poor skin turgor
- Delirium
- Orthostatic hypotension
- Decreased urine output
- Nightmares

- Increased temperature
- Lethargy
- Constipation
- Decreased jugular venous pressure for all of the manifestations

(Ellershaw et al., 1995; Fainsinger & Bruera, 1995; Kedziera, 2001; MacDonald, 1998; Periera & Bruera, 1997)

Management

A. General measures: Hydration is accomplished by parenteral infusions ($$) and hypodermoclysis ($) (subcutaneous administration of fluids) when fluid replacement by mouth requires augmentation (Fainsinger & Bruera, 1995).

B. Death is not imminent.
1. When the decision is made to hydrate a patient, various options are available.
2. Patients should always be encouraged to take oral fluids.
3. Hypodermoclysis provides easier access; sites can last up to a week and can be easily discontinued. If there is poor subcutaneous absorption, healthcare providers may add 150 u hyaluronidase (Wydase®) to 1,000 cc normal saline. If site is reddened and the patient is not uncomfortable, continue with infusion (Ellershaw et al., 1995; Fainsinger & Bruera, 1995; Kedziera, 2001; MacDonald, 1998; Periera & Bruera, 1997).

C. Death is imminent.
1. If the patient is close to death, it may not be necessary to hydrate.
2. However, adjust the doses of medications to prevent drug metabolite accumulation (Periera & Bruera, 1997).

Patient Outcomes

A. Maintainenance of optimal hydration status

B. Avoidance of adverse effects of dehydration when possible

Professional Competencies

A. Perform ongoing assessment to evaluate the patient's physical and cognitive status.

B. Initiate medication dose reduction in the actively dying patient to prevent metabolite toxicity.

C. Administer alternative hydration when appropriate.

D. Evaluate effectiveness of interventions and adjust as appropriate.

References

Ellershaw, J., Sutcliffe, J., & Saunders, C. (1995). Dehydration and the dying patient. *Journal of Pain and Symptom Management, 10*(3), 192–197.

Fainsinger, R., & Bruera, E. (1995). The management of dehydration in terminally ill patients. *Journal of Palliative Care, 10*(3), 55–59.

Kedziera, P. (2001). Hydration, thirst, and nutrition. In B.R. Ferrell & N. Coyle (Eds.), *Textbook of palliative nursing* (pp. 156–163). New York: Oxford University Press.

MacDonald, N. (1998). Ethical issues in dehydration and nutrition. In E. Bruera & R.K. Portenoy (Eds.), *Topics in palliative care* (Vol. 2) (pp. 153–169). New York: Oxford University Press.

Periera, J., & Bruera, E. (1997). *The Edmonton aid to palliative care*. Edmonton, Canada: University of Alberta.

Delirium/Acute Confusion

Howard Smith, MD

Definition

Delirium can be defined as an acute confusional state resulting from global impairment of mental function. This contrasts from dementia, which follows a predictable chronic loss of cognition. Delirium generally occurs fairly rapidly (hours, days) and presents as disorientation, especially to time and place, and can fluctuate over a period of time (e.g., may get worse at night, as in "sundown syndrome"). Although usually described as a transient and potentially reversible disorder of cognition, delirium usually occurs in the last hours or days of life as an irreversible terminal event (Lawlor, Fainsinger, & Bruera, 2000).

Pathophysiology/Etiology

Advanced illness is a risk factor for both confusion and delirium with multifactorial etiologies. Frequent causes of delirium include medications such as psychotropics, chemotherapy, corticosteroids, opiates, anticholinergics, and antiemetics. Drug toxicity (e.g., digoxin, quinidine, lithium, antidepressants) may be responsible for roughly one-third of all cases of delirium (Lawlor et al., 2000). Other contributing factors can include fluid and electrolyte imbalances, hepatic or renal dysfunction, ischemia or hypoxia, and systemic or specific infections (Lawlor et al.). Unmanaged pain (delirium occasionally can be a contributing factor to "crescendo" pain) (Coyle, Breitbart, Weaver, & Portenoy, 1994) or other persistent symptoms accompanying advanced pathophysiologic changes resulting from malignant and nonmalignant disease can cause delirium.

Manifestations

* Sudden change in cognition
* Restlessness/agitation

- Impaired cognition/reduced sensorium
- Hallucinations
- Sleep/wake cycle disruption
- Memory loss/attention deficit

(Lawlor et al., 2000; Storey, 1994)

Management

A. General measures
1. Assess and treat reversible causes, such as hydration and electrolyte replacement.
2. Provide a calm and reassuring environment, including the use of orientation measures such as a clock, calendar, and familiar photographs.
3. Avoid excessive sensory stimulus by providing a quiet, relaxed, and safe setting.
4. Do not consider making any abrupt changes for the patient during this time; maintain consistency with familiar people and surroundings.
5. Pharmacologic interventions for delirium should begin with a review of all trialed and current medications. Discontinuing or tapering medications may prove useful to reduce changes in cognition. If patient is dehydrated, it may be necessary to hydrate with normal saline solution ($).
6. Consider switching opiates if patient is demonstrating metabolite toxicity.
7. Taper anxiolytics, especially benzodiazepines, because of their long-acting metabolites that can contribute to delirium.
8. Evaluate for potential substance withdrawal and treat if necessary.
9. Haloperidol (Haldol®) ($) is considered the medication of choice. Use a sliding scale from 0.5–2 mg q 4–6 hours po/sq.
10. Chlorpromazine (Thorazine®) ($) may be used if haloperidol is ineffective. Chlorpromazine is more sedating. Titrate on a sliding scale from 10–100 mg q 6–8 hours po/pr.
11. Midazolam (Versed®) ($$) also may be considered but only in severe delirium while pursuing treatments of reversible causes.
12. Newer medications, such as risperidone (Risperdal®) ($$) (Sipahimalani & Masand, 1997) and olanzapine (Zyprexa®) ($$) (Sipahimalani & Masand, 1998), have demonstrated effectiveness in the treatment of delirium and should be considered in sequential trials to promote comfort.

Patient Outcomes

A. Optimal cognition is maintained until death.

B. Safety is maintained during episodes of delirium.

Professional Competencies

A. Assess, evaluate, and treat reversible causes of delirium.

B. Identify reversible factors that contribute to delirium (e.g., medication toxicity, dehydration, electrolyte imbalances, disease-related entities) and treat accordingly (Storey, 1994).

C. Taper and titrate medications to produce optimal results.

D. Maintain a calm and consistently safe environment for the patient.

References

Coyle, N., Breitbart, W., Weaver, J., & Portenoy, R. (1994). Delirium as a contributing factor to "crescendo" pain: Three case reports. *Journal of Pain and Symptom Management, 9,* 44–47.

Lawlor, P., Fainsinger, R., & Bruera, E. (2000). Delirium at the end of life: Critical issues in clinical practice and research. *JAMA, 284,* 2427–2429.

Sipahimalani, A., & Masand, P. (1997). Use of risperidone in delirium: Case reports. *Annals of Clinical Psychiatry, 9,* 105–107.

Sipahimalani, A., & Masand, P. (1998). Olanzapine in the treatment of delirium. *Psychosomatics, 39,* 422–430.

Storey, P. (1994). *Primer of palliative care.* Gainesville, FL: Academy of Hospice and Palliative Medicine.

Depression

William Breitbart, MD, E. Duke Dickerson, MSc, PhD,
John L. Shuster, Jr., MD, Jeffery P. Henderson, MS,
Joshua M. Cox, RPh, and Mellar Davis, MD, FCCP

Definition

A mood state that spans a continuum from minor alterations in mood to pathologic loss of the ability to cope with life. It is recognized as the most common
mental health problem in palliative care.

Pathophysiology/Etiology

Advanced illness can produce many of the somatic signs and symptoms (e.g.,
fatigue, loss of energy) seen in depression. As a result, the presence of those symptoms is not conclusive for a diagnosis of a depressive disorder. A diagnosis of
depression in advanced cancer is based on psychologic or cognitive symptoms
(e.g., worthlessness, hopelessness, excessive guilt, suicidal ideation) of major depression (American Psychiatric Association, 1994). Conventional treatment leads
to a positive response in more than 80% of cases. However, evidence suggests that
many cases of depression are not diagnosed (Breitbart, Chochinov, & Passik, 1998).

Manifestations

- Depressed mood reported or observed to be distinctly different from normal
  mood variations and causes suffering, distress, or dysfunction
- Depressed mood that is present most of the day for at least two weeks
- Sometimes distinguishing between the presence of other symptoms (e.g., sleep
  disturbance, loss of weight/appetite, impaired concentration, psychomotor re-
  tardation, loss of interest, feelings of guilt, fatigue or loss of energy, suicidal
  ideations or thoughts of death) that cannot be attributed to the physical disease
  is difficult.
- Sadness may be part of a normal adjustment reaction and require counseling
  and social support rather than medication. Symptoms that meet diagnostic

criteria should be treated with antidepressant medications, augmented by counseling and social contact.

Management

Life expectancy is a major determinant to which pharmacotherapeutic agents will be used in the treatment of depression. The most commonly used therapeutic drug classes are tricylic antidepressants (TCAs), selective serotonin reuptake inhibitors (SSRIs), and psychostimulants (see Table 1). TCAs and SSRIs generally take a minimum of two weeks to provide therapeutic benefit for depression and are not appropriate for patients with a life expectancy of less than four weeks (i.e., most American hospice patients).

A. Death is not imminent.
   1. For patients with a life expectancy of more than four weeks, the choice of antidepressant will be based upon the individual patient's medical profile.
   2. Table 1 can be used as a guide for the various classes of antidepressant agents (Esper & Redman, 1999).

B. Death is imminent: For patients with a life expectancy of four weeks or less, a psychostimulant (e.g., dextroamphetamine [Dexedrine®], methylphenidate [Ritalin®]) generally is recommended.
   1. The main advantage of psychostimulants is a rapid onset of antidepressant action compared to TCAs and SSRIs.

Table 1. Classifications of Antidepressant Agents

Classification	Advantages	Side effects
Selective serotonin reuptake inhibitors (SSRIs) ($$–$$$) • Sertraline (Zoloft®) • Paroxetine (Paxil®) • Fluoxetine (Prozac®)	Fewer side effects than TCAs Fewer drug interactions than TCAs Decreased risk of overdose	Mild nausea Headache Somnolence Appetite suppression Brief episodes of anxiety
Tricyclic antidepressants (TCAs) ($–$$) • Amitriptyline (Elavil®) • Imipramine (Tofranil®) • Nortriptyline (Pamelor®)	First choice in patients with peripheral symptoms (insomnia, incontinence)	Sedation Cardiac arrhythmias Anticholinergic effects
Miscellaneous agents • Mirtazapine (Remeron®) ($$$) • Dextroamphetamine (Dexedrine®) ($) • Methylphenidate (Ritalin®) ($$)	No anticholinergic, adrenergic, or typical SSRI side effects Can decrease fatigue and promote increased sense of well-being	Somnolence Increased appetite Constipation Tachycardia Nervousness Insomnia

2. There is a low incidence of side effects, the augmentation of opioid analgesia, the reversing of opiate-induced sedation, and an enhancement of appetite in cachexic patients, which add to the usefulness of psycho-stimulants in palliative care (Brannon & Stone, 1999).

3. An effective starting dose of methylphenidate is 5 mg po in the morning. If no evidence of adverse reaction is apparent, an additional dose of 5 mg may be administered 4 hours later (e.g., 8 am and noon). Dextroamphetamine is dosed once daily, starting at 5 mg po in the morning. A therapeutic effect may become apparent within two days. Maximum doses are 40–60 mg/day.

4. Because of stimulant effects, every effort should be made to avoid adminis-tration in the late afternoon or evening hours (Shuster, Chochinov, & Green-berg, 2000).

Patient Outcomes

A. Resolution of target symptoms

B. Relief of suffering, distress, and dysfunction related to mood

Professional Competencies

A. Differentiation is made between sadness, situational depression, and a depres-sive disorder.

B. Once identified, depression is treated based on the patient's general medical condition and life expectancy.

C. Adjustments are made in antidepressant dosing that reflect knowledge of the pharmacodynamics of antidepressant agents.

D. The treatment plan is evaluated and modified for optimal patient outcomes.

Measurement Instruments

A. Hospital Anxiety and Depression Scale (HADS) (Zigmond & Snaith, 1983)
   1. Can be useful in identifying depressive disorders in patients with advanced illness
   2. HADS, a 14-item self-rating questionnaire with subscales for depression and anxiety, has been demonstrated to be an effective tool for screening depres-sive disorders in patients with cancer (Derogatis & Melisaratos, 1983).

B. Distress thermometer (a visual analog scale to measure nonspecific distress)

C. Prime-MD Mood Module (structured interview allows accurate diagnosis of mood disorders in less than five minutes) (Spitzer et al., 1994)

References

American Psychiatric Association. (1994). *Diagnostic and statistical manual of mental disorders* (4th ed.). Washington, DC: Author.

Brannon, G., & Stone, K. (1999). The use of mirtazapine in a patient with chronic pain. *Journal of Pain and Symptom Management, 18,* 382–385.

Breitbart, W., Chochinov, H., & Passik, S. (1998). Psychiatric aspects of palliative care. In D. Doyle, G.W.C. Hanks, & N. MacDonald (Eds.), *Oxford textbook of palliative medicine* (2nd ed.) (pp. 933–954). New York: Oxford University Press.

Derogatis, L., & Melisaratos, N. (1983). The Brief Symptom Inventory (BSI): An introductory report. *Psychological Medicine, 13,* 595–605.

Esper, P., & Redman, B. (1999). Supportive care, pain management and quality of life in advance prostate cancer. *Urologic Clinics of North America, 26,* 375–390.

Shuster, J.L., Chochinov, H.M., & Greenberg, D.B. (2000). Psychiatric aspects and psychopharmacologic strategies in palliative care. In A. Stoudemire, B.F. Fogel, & D.B. Greenberg (Eds.), *Psychiatric care of the medical patient* (Vol. 2) (pp. 315–327). New York: Oxford University Press.

Spitzer, R.L., Williams, J.B., Kroenke, K., Linzer, M., deGruy, F.V., Hahn, S.R., Brody, D., & Johnson, J.G. (1994). Utility of a new procedure for diagnosing mental disorders in primary care. The PRIME-MD 1000 study. *JAMA, 272,* 1749–1756.

Zigmond, A., & Snaith, R. (1983). The hospital anxiety and depression scale. *Acta Psychiatrica Scandinavica, 67,* 361–370.

Diarrhea

Beth Cohen, RNC, ARNP, MSN

Definition

Diarrhea is the elimination of several loose or watery bowel movements that interfere with the body's fluid and electrolyte balance.

Pathophysiology/Etiology

Chronically ill patients may experience mild diarrhea lasting only a day or two or it may be severe and often debilitating. Causes include infection, chronic inflammatory conditions (colitis, Crohn's disease), food/lactose intolerances, emotional stress, parasites, gastrointestinal bleeding, and medications. The result can have a profound effect on the patient's quality of life, leading to skin breakdown, dehydration, malnutrition, and severe weight loss (Greif & Golden, 1994; Sande & Volberding, 1999).

Manifestations

- Fatigue
- Weakness
- Hemorrhoids
- Abdominal pain/cramping
- Fecal incontinence
- Fever
- Decreased appetite (anorexia)
- Dehydration
- Malaise
- Obstruction
- Fluid/electrolyte imbalance

Management

A. Death is not imminent.

1. Antidiarrheal medication ($–$$)—Available in liquid and pill form, by prescription or over the counter. Beneficial to decrease the number of stools per day, thereby decreasing the risk of dehydration, fatigue, electrolyte imbalance, and hemorrhoids. Side effects can include nausea, vomiting, constipation, abdominal bloating, flatulence, and unpleasant taste (Doughty, 2000; Hodgson & Kizior, 2001). Infection, impaction, and *Clostridium difficile* should be ruled out prior to initiating these medications (Paganar & Paganar, 1998).

2. Psyllium products ($)—Can improve stool consistency (by absorbing water), therefore decreasing the "watery" nature of the stool. They do not reduce stool volume but assist in maintaining continence (Doughty; Hodgson & Kizior).

3. Hydration ($–$$$)—Used to prevent dehydration and electrolyte imbalance (Greif & Golden, 1994; Sande & Volberding, 1999)

4. Skin care ($–$$)—Steps must be taken to prevent skin breakdown, including avoiding the use of diapers, keeping skin clean with soap and water, and protecting the skin with an over-the-counter cream or ointment that will provide a moisture barrier (either petroleum-based, zinc oxide based, or dimethicone-based). A skin barrier powder and alcohol-free sealant may be used covered with a moisture barrier ointment, or absorptive skin barrier paste may be used for treatment of denuded skin. Paste must be applied in a thick layer, and only the top soiled layer should be removed when cleaning the patient. New paste should be reapplied on top of the old. Use of a perineal cleanser may help removal of the paste without trauma to the skin (Doughty).

5. Fecal incontinence collectors ($–$$)—Almost always able to use in men, in women feasibility is determined by the skin bridge between the anus and vagina. Severely denuded skin will be difficult to pouch. Area may need to be shaved prior to applying the pouch. Skin preparation with application of a protective barrier solution is necessary. Primarily used on bed-bound patients (Doughty).

6. Dietary guidelines—Dietary alterations to help decrease diarrhea may include following a BRAT (banana, rice, applesauce, tea) diet or avoiding spicy, greasy, or gas-producing foods (Greif & Golden).

B. Death is imminent.
   1. Attempts should be made, if appropriate, to treat diarrhea. Keeping the patient clean, dry, and comfortable is the priority.
   2. Use medications as previously described.

Patient Outcomes

A. Control of diarrhea

B. Relief of diarrhea-associated symptoms (e.g., fatigue, dehydration) and prevention of diarrhea-associated problems

Professional Competencies

A. Identify abnormal bowel patterns early to prevent further complications, such as impaction, dehydration, and fatigue.

B. Evaluate the effectiveness of interventions by regularly assessing bowel patterns, and modify the plan of care accordingly. Prevent the complications associated with frequent diarrhea.

References

Doughty, D. (2000, November). *Challenges in geriatric nursing.* Unpublished handout provided at the Wound, Ostomy, Continence Nursing in the Geriatric Population Seminar, Boca Raton, FL.

Greif, J., & Golden, B.A. (1994). *AIDS care at home.* New York: John Wiley & Sons.

Hodgson, B., & Kizior, R. (2001). *Saunders nursing drug handbook 2001.* Philadelphia: W.B. Saunders.

Paganar, K.D., & Paganar, T.J. (1998). *Mosby's manual of diagnostics and laboratory tests.* St. Louis, MO: Mosby.

Sande, M., & Volberding, P. (1999). *Medical management of AIDS* (6th ed.). St. Louis, MO: Mosby.

Dysphagia

Pamela Spencer, BA, MSN, MSN, FNP

Definition

Dysphagia is difficultly in swallowing. It specifically refers to the sensation of food or liquids being hindered in the normal passage from the mouth to the stomach (Twycross, 1997).

Pathophysiology/Etiology

Patients with chronic esophageal or oropharyngeal conditions often develop dysphagia. The cause is multifactorial and includes motor impairment or mechanical obstruction of the esophagus, either intrinsically from narrowing due to tumors, strictures, webs or rings or extrinsically through compression of the esophagus from causes such as mediastinal tumors and vascular anomalies (Twycross, 1997; Woodruff, 1997). The buccal phase of dysphagia is identified when food is voluntarily pushed backward by the tongue and palate; this can occur as a result of infection, radiation, or chemotherapy. The pharyngeal phase of dysphagia occurs when the swallowing reflex initiates glottis closure; this can occur as a result of infection, radiation, or surgery that has complicated the ability to swallow (Twycross). The esophageal phase of dysphagia (when food is passed down the esophagus by reflex peristalsis) can become limited by infection, radiation, gastric reflux, surgery, fibrosis/stricture, or anxiety.

Manifestations
Oropharyngeal Dysphagia
- Repeated attempts to initiate swallowing
- Nasal regurgitation of liquids
- Coughing while eating
- Foods sticking in the throat

Esophageal Dysphagia

- Foods "stick" after being swallowed
- Chronic heartburn and achalasia
- Mechanical obstruction: Patients have difficulty with solids only
- Chest pain
- Diffuse esophageal spasms

(Twycross, 1997; Woodruff, 1997)

Management

A. Death is not imminent.
   1. Buccal and pharyngeal dysphagia call for feeding education, which includes assistance and direction on positioning techniques, dietary advice, and enteral nutrition (Twycross, 1997).
   2. Treat and avoid causative or aggravating factors, including medications, dehydration, dry atmosphere, smoking, and anxiety.
   3. Obstructing tumors—surgery, laser resection, or radiotherapy
   4. Extrinsic compression—corticosteroids or radiotherapy
   5. Neuromuscular coordination—corticosteroids or radiotherapy
   6. Stomatitis, pharyngitis, xerostomia ($–$$)—nystatin Swish and Swallow®; fluoride gels and rinses; sialogogues, such as bethanechol (Urecholine®), neostigmine methylsulfate (Prostigmin®), and pilocarpine (Salagen®); pain relief with local anesthetics (2% xylocaine [Lidocaine®]; viscous, nonsteroidal anti-inflammatory medications; salicylates; and mucosal protective agents (Skidmore-Roth, 1999; Twycross; Woodruff, 1997).
   7. If complete obstruction remains present, drooling can lead to aspiration and may require anticholingeric medications to reduce salivary flow ($).
   8. Antiulcer medications are considered when esophageal dysphagia is present ($–$$).
   9. Chronic stricture requires dilation ($$), chemotherapy, or radiation ($$$).

B. Death is imminent.
   1. Patients with oropharyngeal dysphagia should be managed conservatively, with dietary manipulation.
   2. Patients with esophageal dysphagia should be managed symptomatically (Twycross, 1997; Woodruff, 1997).
      a) Evaluate positioning changes.
      b) Topical anesthetics, combined antacids, and dietary manipulation are helpful ($–$$).
      c) Opiates should be considered if pain is present ($–$$$).

Patient Outcomes

A. Plan of care understood and agreed upon

B. Relief of dysphagia and associated symptoms

Professional Competencies

A. Determine the probable etiology of dysphagia when possible.

B. Interventions are based upon preferences and expected survival.

C. Facilitate referral for treatment of dysphagia as appropriate.

D. Provide pharmacologic interventions based upon the individual and the extent of the disease process.

E. Perform ongoing assessment and evaluation of the effectiveness of specific interventions.

References

Skidmore-Roth, L. (1999). *Mosby's 1999 nursing drug reference.* St. Louis, MO: Mosby.

Twycross, R. (1997). Dysphagia. In R. Twycross (Ed.), *Symptom management in advanced cancer* (2nd ed.) (pp. 174–181). London: Radcliffe Medical Press.

Woodruff, R. (1997). *Symptom control in advanced cancer.* Melbourne, Australia: Asperula Publisher.

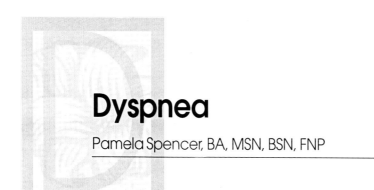

Dyspnea

Pamela Spencer, BA, MSN, BSN, FNP

Definition

Dyspnea is defined as an uncomfortable awareness of breathing. Dyspnea is often described as breathlessness or severe shortness of breath and is estimated to occur in 50%–70% of patients at the end of life (Pereira & Bruera, 1997).

Pathophysiology/Etiology

Several pathophysiologic processes contribute to dyspnea. The most important of these is the increased effort to breathe, which accompanies many different diseases that interfere with airflow (McDermott, 2000). Advanced illnesses that prevent airflow include chronic obstructive pulmonary diseases, such as asthma and emphysema. Changes in pulmonary compliance that interfere with the workload of breathing include interstitial fibrosis, congestive heart failure, intrinsic respiratory muscle weakness, or hyperinflation. Airway obstruction resulting from tumors can include the trachea, larynx, thyroid, mediastinum, and bronchus and tracheoesophageal fistula. Dyspnea inhibits the patient's ability to engage in normal activities, which can lead to social isolation and a decreased quality of life (Kuebler, 2002; McDermott; Pereira & Bruera, 1997).

Manifestations

- Tachypnea
- Digital clubbing
- Pallor
- Confusion
- Cyanosis
- Coughing
- Use of accessory muscles

- Restlessness
- Memory or concentration difficulties
- Tachycardia
- Nasal flaring
- Crackles/wheezing
- Intercostal retractions

(Kuebler, 2002; McDermott, 2000; Pereira & Bruera, 1997)

Management

A. Death is not imminent (Kuebler, 2002; Pereira & Bruera, 1997).
   1. Nonpharmacologic interventions, including breathing techniques (See Complementary Therapies.)
   2. Bronchodilators ($)—nebulized: ipratropium (Atrovent®), albuterol (Proventil®), isoproterenol (Isuprel®), or metaproterenol (Alupent®). Systemic bronchodilators: theophylline (Theo-Dur®)
   3. Corticosteroids ($)—nebulized: beclomethasone (Beclovent®). Systemic: dexamethasone (Decadron®), prednisone (Deltasone®), or methylprednisolone (Medrol®)
   4. Opiates ($–$$$)—Morphine used orally (immediate release or liquid), subcutaneously, sublingually ($), or in the form of nebulized inhalation therapy
   5. Anxiolytics—benzodiazepines ($$) and phenothiazines ($)
   6. Diuretics ($)—furosemide (Lasix®), spironolactone (Aldactone®), and chlorothiazide (Diuril®) should only be considered if the patient is not hypovolemic.
   7. Blood transfusions ($$)—treatment of anemia
   8. Erythropoietin ($$$)—restoration
   9. Radiation therapy or chemotherapy ($$$$)

B. Death is imminent (Kuebler, 1996, 2002; Pereira & Bruera, 1997).
   1. Anticholinergics ($)—scopolamine, atropine
   2. Oxygen ($$)—nasal cannula if possible to improve patient comfort
   3. Morphine (see medications above)
   4. Terminal sedation if needed

Patient Outcomes

A. Uses breathing techniques or medications to minimize dyspnea

B. Able to perform activities that are of importance

C. Able to breathe without discomfort

Professional Competencies

A. Treat underlying etiology as possible.

B. Provide interventions based upon disease trajectory (i.e., palliative versus aggressive).

C. Assess effectiveness of interventions regularly and modify the treatment plan to promote optimal outcomes.

D. Tailor patient and family education to their literacy level and provide comfort at home.

References

Kuebler, K. (1996). *Hospice and palliative care clinical practice protocol: Dyspnea.* Pittsburgh: Hospice Nurses Association.

Kuebler, K. (2002). Dyspnea. In K. Kuebler, P. Berry, & D. Heidrich (Eds.), *End-of-life care: Clinical practice guidelines for advanced practice nursing* (pp. 301–316). Philadelphia: W.B. Saunders.

McDermott, M.K. (2000). Dyspnea. In D. Camp-Sorrell & R.A. Hawkins (Eds.), *Clinical manual for the oncology advanced practice nurse.* Pittsburgh: Oncology Nursing Press.

Pereira, J., & Bruera, E. (1997). *The Edmonton aid to palliative care.* Alberta, Canada: University of Alberta, Division of Palliative Care.

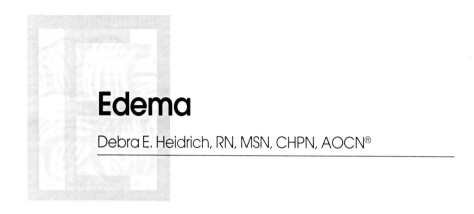

Edema

Debra E. Heidrich, RN, MSN, CHPN, AOCN®

Definition

Edema is the abnormal accumulation of fluid in the intracellular spaces.

Pathophysiology/Etiology

Edema is the result of a number of pathophysiologic alterations that lead to either fluid overload or failure to excrete fluids. In palliative care, common causes of edema are cardiac, renal, or hepatic failure; hypoalbuminemia; inappropriate antidiuretic hormone secretion (SIADH); and immobility. (Small cell lung cancer is the most common cause of SIADH.) Administration of enteral or parenteral fluids in the presence of renal or cardiac compromise will lead to edema. Medications, such as corticosteroids and some hormonal agents, will contribute to edema. Edema interferes with the normal exchange of nutrition and excretion within cells, leading to an increased risk of tissue breakdown (Twycross, 1997; Waller & Caroline, 2000).

Manifestations

- Swollen extremities with or without pitting
- Pale and cool skin
- Discomfort in edematous tissue
- Tissue breakdown
- Weeping of skin
- Dyspnea

With SIADH, the following symptoms are seen.
- Fatigue or lethargy
- Muscle cramps
- Nausea
- Headache
- Severe: confusion, seizures, or coma

Management

A. Death is not imminent.

1. Encourage exercise, as tolerated, to improve circulation. Walking, active or passive range of motion, and isometric exercises are helpful (Waller & Caroline, 2000).

2. Encourage use of compression stockings if the patient is active. Bedridden patients do not benefit by using compression stockings ($$) (Waller & Caroline).

3. Elevate edematous extremities to the level of the heart or above.

4. Consider pros and cons of using diuretic therapy. Do not use diuretics unless edema is causing discomfort or physiologic compromise.

    a) Furosemide (Lasix®) ($), 20–40 mg po q/day, or spironolactone (Aldactone®) ($), 100 mg po q/day, may be helpful. Dosages may be increased if not effective after several days (Waller & Caroline).

    b) Administer diuretics in the morning.

    c) Evaluate patient's ability to reach bathroom or bedside commode quickly and the energy expenditure this requires. Catheterization may be necessary to promote comfort and save energy for other activities valued by the patient.

5. Dietary changes are rarely helpful in the palliative care setting. If patient feels like eating, encourage high-protein foods. Fluid and sodium restrictions are not appropriate.

6. Decrease or discontinue enteral or parenteral fluids if they are contributing to edema.

7. Treat the symptomatic hyponatremia of SIADH.

8. Demeclocycline (Declomycin®) ($$)—300 mg po bid interferes with the ADH effect on renal tubules and promotes fluid excretion by the kidneys (Bower, Brazil, & Coombes, 1998; Twycross, 1997).

9. Restriction of free fluid intake to < 1 liter/day may be helpful. In the palliative care setting, a patient's fluid intake often is < 1 liter without any stated restrictions.

10. Urea 30 g ($$) dissolved in 100 cc orange juice po is sometimes used as an osmotic diuretic. Administration of urea eliminates the need for any fluid restriction. Although orange juice helps to mask the taste of urea, patients may find this medication objectionable (Bower et al.; Twycross).

11. IV infusion of 0.9%–3% saline, in combination with diuretics ($$$), is reserved for severe hyponatremia, when the patient's functional status is likely to improve with treatment. If functional status is not likely to improve, this intervention should not be used in the palliative care setting (Twycross).

12. Protect skin with moisturizers, gentle handling, and appropriate positioning and support to minimize pressure.

B. Death is imminent.
1. Continue to provide excellent skin care.
2. Elevate edematous extremities if this promotes comfort.
3. Discontinue diuretics unless patient is catheterized. As death approaches, assess for need to continue diuretics.
4. Discontinue enteral or parenteral fluids if they are causing edema.

Patient Outcomes

A. Maintenance of comfort

B. Achievement of optimal functional status

C. Absence of skin breakdown

Professional Competencies

A. Individuals at risk for edema are identified and regularly assessed for signs of edema.

B. Measures to prevent edema are instituted when possible.

C. Effectiveness of interventions is evaluated regularly, and the intervention plan is modified, with a goal of promoting comfort and preventing complications (versus resolution of edema).

D. Caregivers are instructed on the appropriate administration of medications, positioning techniques, care and inspection of skin, and signs and symptoms to report to healthcare professionals.

References

Bower, M., Brazil, L., & Coombes, R.C. (1998). Endocrine and metabolic complications of advanced cancer. In D. Doyle, G.W.C. Hanks, & N. MacDonald (Eds.), *Oxford textbook of palliative medicine* (2nd ed.) (pp. 709–725). New York: Oxford University Press.

Twycross, R. (1997). *Symptom management in advanced cancer* (2nd ed.). Abingdon, England: Radcliffe Medical Press.

Waller, A., & Caroline, N.L. (2000). *Handbook of palliative care in cancer.* Boston: Butterworth-Heinemann.

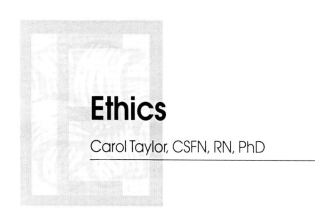

Ethics

Carol Taylor, CSFN, RN, PhD

Definition

Ethics is a systematic inquiry into the principles of right and wrong conduct, of virtue and vice, and of good and evil as they relate to conduct. Ethics also may be defined as the study of who we ought to be in light of who we say we are (Fletcher, 1997).

Specific Issues Related to Palliative Care

Ethics raises questions about how we should to live (and die) and why. Recently the five-year, $25 million SUPPORT study, designed to identify and correct problems associated with end-of-life care, demonstrated that many of us are not dying well. After intervention, no improvements were seen on any of the following outcomes.

- Physician-patient communication (37% of the control patients and 40% of intervention patients discussed cardiopulmonary resuscitation [CPR] preferences)
- Incidence or timing of do not resuscitate orders
- Physicians' knowledge of patients' preferences about CPR
- Days spent in the intensive care unit
- Use of mechanical ventilation
- Days comatose before death
- Level of reported pain
- Use of hospital resources

Among the more than 4,000 patients who died in the postintervention phase, 10% received more aggressive care than they wanted, and 40% had severe pain most of the time (Moskowitz & Nelson, 1995).

Ethics asks what it means to die well and what society and medical institutions need to change to help people die well. Ethical issues at the end of life thus include human dignity concerns, diminished patient autonomy (fear of not being "allowed" to die or of being forced to die before one is ready), issues concerning appropriate pain and symptom management and related interventions (e.g., terminal sedation), guidelines for withholding and withdrawing life-sustaining treatment, assisted suicide, and direct euthanasia (Quill, 1993; Quill, Lee, & Nunn, 2000).

Ethical Theories

Different theories raise different questions, as the examples below demonstrate.

- Which alternative would help one develop and maintain valuable traits of character (i.e., be a person of courage or compassion)? *The Virtue Approach*
- Which alternative would lead to the best overall consequences? *The Utilitarian Approach*
- Which alternative best respects and protects the moral rights of individuals? *The Rights Approach*
- Which alternative treats all parties in a fair or just manner? *The Fairness (or Justice) Approach*
- Which alternative best promotes the common good? *The Common Good Approach*
- Which alternative is most responsive to the individualized needs of each of the people involved—those with unique narratives and plans? What are my fiduciary responsibilities to involved individuals? *The Care-Based Approach*

Principle-Based Ethics

The principle-based approach to doing bioethics offers specific action guides for practice (Beauchamp & Childress, 2001) (see Table 1).

Table 1. Principle-Based Ethics

Principle	Moral Rule	Implications for Practice
Autonomy (self-determination)	Respect the rights of patients or their surrogates to make healthcare decisions.	Provide the information and support patients and families need to make the decision that is right for them; at times, this may mean collaborating with other members of the healthcare team to advocate for the patient.
Nonmaleficence	Avoid causing harm.	Do not seek to inflict harm and prevent harm or risk of harm whenever possible.
Beneficence	Benefit the patient and balance benefits against risks and harms.	Commit yourself to actively promote the patient's benefit (health and well-being). Be sensitive to the fact that individuals (patients, family members, and professional caregivers) may identify benefits and harms differently. A benefit to one may be a burden to another.

(Continued on next page)

Table 1. Principle-Based Ethics (Continued)

Principle	Moral Rule	Implications for Practice
Justice	Give each his or her due; act fairly.	Always seek to distribute the benefits, risks, and costs of nursing care justly. This may involve recognizing subtle instances of bias and discrimination.
Fidelity	Keep promises.	Be faithful to the promise you made to the public to be competent and willing to use your competence to benefit the patients entrusted to your care. Never abandon a patient entrusted to your care without first providing for his or her needs.

Care-Based Approach

The healthcare professional-patient relationship is central to the care-based approach, which directs attention to the "particulars" of individual patients who are viewed within the context of their life narrative. How a healthcare professional handles encounters with a patient or colleague is a matter of ethical significance. Ethics is not reduced to a decision to withhold or withdraw life-sustaining treatment. Characteristics of the care perspective include

- Centrality of the caring relationship
- Promotion of the dignity and respect of patients as people
- Attention to the particulars about individual patients
- Cultivation of responsiveness to others and professional responsibility
- A redefinition of fundamental moral skills should include virtues like kindness, attentiveness, empathy, compassion, and reliability.

Codes of Ethics/Ethical Directives

Healthcare professionals should be familiar with (a) the code of ethics regulating their professional practice, (b) specific codes of conduct or ethical directives of employing institutions (e.g., religious directives), and (c) pertinent legislation and precedent-setting case norms that offer ethical guidance.

Strategies to Promote Ethics in Palliative Care

As patients and families struggle with end-of-life care and treatment decisions, they are increasingly looking to healthcare professionals for information, advice, and support. Patients have a legally and morally protected right to consent to and to refuse any and all indicated medical therapies. The following interventions can be helpful in promoting quality palliative care.

A. Foster excellent communication among the patient, patient's family, and professional caregiving team.

B. Develop a culture within the institution that supports ethical practice and holds all parties accountable.
    1. Collaborative practice and guidelines for reporting incompetent, unethical, or illegal practice
    2. Strong (and enforced) policies on informed decision making, advance care planning, withholding and withdrawing treatment, do not resuscitate orders, and comfort measures only orders.

C. Develop ethics resources: mentors, ethics consult service, institutional ethics committees.

Patient Outcomes

A. Ethical uncertainty, dilemma, or distress on the part of patients and their families and healthcare professionals is identified and resolved.

B. The ethical integrity of all parties is protected.

Professional Competencies

A. Demonstrate clinical competence.

B. Demonstrate actions that advance the best interests of the patients.

C. Hold oneself and one's colleagues accountable for practice.

D. Work collaboratively to advocate for patients, families, and communities.

E. Mediate ethical conflict among the patient, significant others, the healthcare team, and other interested parties.

F. Critique new healthcare technologies and changes in the way healthcare is defined, administered, delivered, and financed related to its potential to influence human well-being.

References

Beauchamp, T.L., & Childress, J.F. (2001). *Principles of biomedical ethics* (5th ed.). New York: Oxford University Press.

Fletcher, J.C. (Ed.). (1997). *Introduction to clinical ethics* (2nd ed.). Frederick, MD: University Publishing Group.

Moskowitz, E.H., & Nelson, J.L. (Eds.). (1995). Dying well in the hospital. The lessons of SUPPORT. *Hastings Center Report, 25*(Suppl. 6), S1–S36.

Quill, T.E. (1993). Doctor, I want to die. Will you help me? *JAMA, 270,* 870–876.

Quill, T.E., Lee, B.C., & Nunn, S. (2000). Palliative treatments of last resort: Choosing the least harmful alternative. *Annals of Internal Medicine, 132,* 488–493.

Family Issues

Karen J. Stanley, RN, MSN, AOCN®, FAAN

Definition

Living with a terminal illness can be likened to the effects caused by a stone being thrown into still waters. Although the patient becomes the focus of the plan of care, those individuals who belong to the immediate circle of family and friends are also deeply affected by the realities of illness.

Specific Issues Related to Palliative Care

A. Familial realization of the severity of illness can be overwhelming.
   1. Family systems suddenly may find themselves confronted with difficult and emotionally painful circumstances that require frequent decision making.
   2. This discomfort may also affect the patients' sense of well-being, as they see their loved ones struggling with their own issues of loss (Bush, 1998).

B. Traditional healthcare systems may not focus on specific family issues.
   1. The primary focus is on patient treatments and diagnostics, leaving family members feeling isolated or helpless when trying to understand what is happening to their loved ones.
   2. It is difficult for family members to ask specific questions when they do not know what questions to ask.

C. Unresolved familial conflict may interfere with effective communication.
   1. Buried, unresolved emotional issues may interfere with effective communication with the patient.
   2. A family member may need to resolve difficult past issues before moving forward with facing an impending loss.

Strategies to Maintain Optimal Family Functioning

A. Evaluate the patient's and family's understanding of the disease process and prognosis.

1. Ongoing assessment and evaluation of what the patient and his or her family understand about the disease process and prognosis will help define specific interventions; bear in mind that the patient may not want additional information.

2. If the patient gives permission, ensure that family members are consistently updated on the patient's prognosis, current status, plan of care, and what to expect as death approaches. This information can relieve anxiety and fear of the unknown, allowing for appropriate planning, provide participation in caregiving needs, and provide an opportunity for family members to describe their expectations.

3. Identify the various developmental stages of individual family members in assessment and planning (Davies, 2000); the differing needs of children and adolescents may require referrals to other members of the interdisciplinary team for individualized intervention.

B. Recognize the interindividuality within each family structure.

1. Many dysfunctional relationships exist within families. This requires assessment of potential unresolved conflicts or general unease among family members. The stressors of illness can exacerbate existing problems, and a careful assessment is essential with an emphasis on using all disciplines to support both the patient and his or her family.

2. Should family members express discomfort with discussing the illness/prognosis with the patient, it may be helpful to assist them with conversational techniques. They can be encouraged to discuss their concerns with each other and to practice what they might say to the patient.

3. Remind family members that these conversations can be very meaningful to the patient (i.e., they allow patients to unburden themselves of fears and anxieties; they relieve the stressors of isolation; they allow unfinished business to be handled; or they provide an opportunity for affection and caring to be expressed) (Stanley, 2001).

C. Identify the decision-making patterns in the family.

1. Although cultural norms and familial patterns may dictate the decision-making role within the family, the clinician should respect the patient's need to be in control. Individuals may choose to make all the decisions while they are able, or they may delegate that responsibility to a specific family member.

2. If an advance directive is in place, it is helpful to discuss both the healthcare preferences and the durable power of attorney in the presence of the patient and family members before a crisis occurs or a difficult decision needs to be made.

D. Understand and acknowledge various coping skills.
1. Assess family coping skills. Individual members may not be prepared to respond in a supportive way.
2. Be alert for warning signs: persistent anger or hostility, illness or health problems, inadequate or inappropriate care giving, and detachment or withdrawal.
3. Acknowledge the emotional difficulties engendered by a terminal illness, offer to listen or facilitate a family conference, and assist with problems that can be solved.
4. Encourage individual strengths and healthy coping skills.
5. Refer family members to community agencies and support groups when appropriate.

Family Outcomes

A. Receive information related to the patient's disease and prognosis based upon what he or she is prepared to hear.

B. Participate in the plan of care based upon the need and desire to do so.

C. Resolve conflict related to past or present issues.

Professional Competencies

A. Provide patient and family-centered palliative care.

B. Encourage and validate open communication.

C. Assess and evaluate patient and family coping skills and developmental issues.

D. Use the interdisciplinary team to support family coping needs.

E. Do not assume that the patient or family will be open to outside intervention— respect individual privacy.

Resources

A. Cancer Survival Toolbox: Free set of audiotapes on communication, decision making, paying for care, and topics for older people. Call 877-TOOLS-4-U or visit the Oncology Nursing Society's Web site: www.ons.org

B. National Family Caregivers Association—10400 Connecticut Ave. #500, Kensington, MD 20895 (800-896-3650) or www.nfcacares.org

C. Rosalynn Carter Institute at Georgia Southwestern State University offers the Caregivers Corner Web site at www.rci.gsw.edu/corner/. The site hosts an active online support group on Mondays at 9 pm ET.

D. "Strength for Caring" focuses on caregiver confidence and competence. Sections include (a) What Is Cancer?, (b) Cancer and the Family, (c) The Role of the Caregiver, and (d) The Caregiver's Role in Symptom Management. Funded by Ortho Biotech. The Oncology Nursing Society Education Cancer Care Issues Team may be contacted for local resources (412-921-7373).

References

Bush, N.J. (1998). Family systems theory: A holistic framework for oncology nursing practice. In R.M. Carroll-Johnson, L.M. Gorman, & N.J. Bush (Eds.), *Psychosocial nursing care along the cancer continuum* (pp. 329–340). Pittsburgh: Oncology Nursing Press.

Davies, B. (2000). Supporting families in palliative care. In B.R. Ferrell & N. Coyle (Eds.), *Textbook of palliative nursing* (pp. 363–373). New York: Oxford University Press.

Stanley, K.J. (2001). Family issues. In R.A. Gates & R.M. Fink (Eds.), *Oncology nursing secrets. Questions and answers about caring for patients with cancer* (2nd ed.) (pp. 534–538). Philadelphia: Hanley & Belfus.

Fatigue

Beth Cohen, RNC, ARNP, MSN

Definition

Often confused with tiredness, fatigue is actually a feeling of sustained exhaustion, weariness, and tiredness. Fatigue is characterized by a daily lack of energy, strength, or endurance. Patients may appear to be lethargic, sleepy, disinterested in their surroundings, and sometimes confused, if severely fatigued. It is a complex phenomenon and is multidimensional, encompassing pathophysiologic, biochemical, and psychologic causes (Barroso, 1999).

Pathophysiology/Etiology

Undeniably, almost all patients with chronic illnesses, such as cancer, will experience fatigue at some point during the continuum of their disease. It can be acute, lasting a month or less, or chronic, lasting from one to six months or longer. Causes include malnutrition; lack of rest or exercise; circulatory disturbances, such as anemia or blood loss; medical conditions, such as hypothyroidism or severe, chronic pain; treatments, such as radiation and chemotherapy; side effects of medications; and tests and procedures that patients undergo. Fatigue also has a psychologic component and occurs when patients are anxious, depressed, or experiencing emotional or physical stress. Overall, fatigue can detrimentally affect patients' quality of life, rendering them unable to enjoy their remaining time (Barroso, 1999; Greif & Golden, 1994).

Manifestations

- Weakness
- Excessive sleep, including naps
- Decreased attention span
- Malaise
- Inability to sleep/insomnia

- Decreased appetite (anorexia)
- Confusion
- Depression
- Pallor

Management

A. General measures
  1. Commonsense interventions, such as providing the patient with a restful, quiet environment
  2. Incorporate rest periods into daily routine.
  3. Space tests or procedures apart by several hours, when able.
  4. Encourage patients to conserve energy for those things they feel are most important.
  5. Provide assistance with activities of daily living, and evaluate ongoing patient safety (Greif & Golden, 1994).

B. Death is not imminent.
  1. Iron supplements ($)
      a) Only beneficial if the fatigue stems from anemia caused by iron deficiency
      b) Available over the counter (in preparations with and without a stool softener) or by prescription
      c) Common side effects include gastrointestinal upset, constipation, and possibly a bad taste in the mouth (Barroso, 1999; Hodgson & Kizior, 2001; Paganar & Paganar, 1998).
  2. Blood transfusion ($$$)—Pre- and post-transfusion evaluation of patient must be performed, with justification of transfusion made before initiating treatment (Barroso; Sande & Volberding, 1999).
  3. Psychologic support ($$)—Referral to a psychologist, counselor, or therapist for assistance in dealing with anxiety, depression, or other emotional issues may be needed (Greif & Golden, 1994).
  4. Nutrition ($–$$)
      a) Consultation with a registered dietitian may be required.
      b) Encourage a well-balanced diet eaten in several small meals with snacks.
      c) Vitamin and nutritional supplements may be prescribed and are available in liquids, snack bars, or puddings (Greif & Golden).

C. Death is imminent.
  1. When the patient is actively dying, attempts to discover the underlying cause of fatigue should be abandoned.
  2. Interventions should be focused on providing comfort resulting from the manifestations of fatigue.
  3. Care should include general measures previously identified, consideration of oxygen as needed, warm clothing, extra blankets, or any measures the patient identifies as comforting.

Patient Outcomes

A. Verbalizes measures to help conserve energy

B. Maintains or regains optimal functional ability until death is imminent

Professional Competencies

A. Identify fatigue and its manifestations in a timely fashion.

B. Determine the appropriateness of aggressive versus palliative interventions.

C. Assess interventions for effectiveness. Modify the treatment plan as appropriate.

Measurement Instruments

A number of instruments currently exists to specifically measure fatigue. Prior to the last decade, the measurement of fatigue was incorporated into other tools, such as the measurement of quality of life. Until recently, fatigue was a neglected topic in medicine and nursing; however, the development of measurement tools specific to fatigue has flourished. The following are just a few examples of fatigue-specific instruments and instruments that incorporate fatigue.

- Visual Analogue Fatigue Scale
- Fatigue Assessment Inventory
- Piper Fatigue Scale—developed for patients with cancer
- Functional Assessment of Cancer Therapy-Anemia (FACT-An)—incorporates the measurement of fatigue
- Functional Assessment of Chronic Illness Therapy (FACIT)—incorporates the measurement of fatigue

References

Barroso, J. (1999). A review of fatigue in people with HIV infection. *Journal of the Association of Nurses in AIDS Care, 10*(5), 42–49.

Greif, J., & Golden, B.A. (1994). *AIDS care at home.* New York: John Wiley & Sons.

Hodgson, B., & Kizior, R. (2001). *Saunders nursing drug handbook 2001.* Philadelphia: W.B. Saunders.

Paganar, K.D., & Paganar, T.J. (1998). *Mosby's manual of diagnostics and laboratory tests.* St. Louis, MO: Mosby.

Sande, M., & Volberding, P. (1999). *Medical management of AIDS* (6th ed.). St. Louis, MO: Mosby.

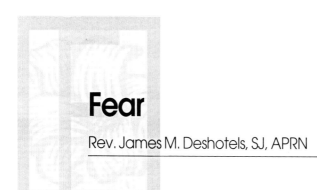

Fear

Rev. James M. Deshotels, SJ, APRN

Definition

Fear is an emotional, physiologic, and behavioral response to a perceived, identified, external threat. Anxiety usually is differentiated from fear by its chronicity and the nature of its object. Fear is the response to a threat, which is known, external, definite, and usually nonconflictual in origin. In anxiety, the object or threat is more likely to be unknown, internal, vague, or arising from psychologic conflict (Amenta, 1997; Friedman, Harrold, & Lynne, 1999; Geist & Jefferson, 1999; Kaplan & Sadock, 1991).

Specific Issues Related to Palliative Care

Fear and anxiety are triggered by the stresses of life, including those involved in the dying process.

Major Fears to Be Addressed

Assessment and evaluation of the cause of fear is very important. Fears and anxieties associated with the dying process include a fear of uncontrolled pain and unbearable suffering, dyspnea and suffocation, and death itself. Other fears will be as unique as the human beings who die (e.g., the patient dying of congestive heart failure whose most pressing concern is who will administer his diabetic wife's insulin after his death).

Fears Specific to Patients and Families

Patients and their families may each experience separate issues of fear, and each must be explored. Patients may have concerns regarding the future of those left behind. Family members may be faced with financial concerns as well as fears related to the actual death experience (Friedman et al., 1999; Geist & Jefferson, 1999; Reimer, Davies, & Martens, 1991; Stiles, 1990).

Strategies to Diminish Fear

A. Patient and family education

Fear of uncontrolled pain, unbearable suffering, dyspnea, and suffocation can be addressed by appropriate education and the use of available pharmacologic and nonpharmacologic interventions. These symptoms can be well controlled but may go uncontrolled when providers and family members fail to overcome fears of their own regarding use of controlled substances and the normal course of dying.

B. Appropriate counseling, spiritual support, and interdisciplinary consultation

The underlying issues of fear require ongoing evaluation and can help the patient deal with fear of death itself. Other fears can be addressed in similar ways. Because fears may be quite realistic and appropriate, this can promote care planning to avoid undesirable outcomes for the patient and significant others (i.e., treatment of dyspnea, pain) (Friedman et al., 1999; Reimer et al., 1991; Stiles, 1990).

Patient Outcomes

A. Eliminates or reduces fear to manageable levels

B. Achieves a realistic perception based upon patient concerns and the disease process

C. Participates in open and caring conversations with loved ones and caregivers (Friedman et al., 1999; Geist & Jefferson, 1999; Reimer et al., 1991; Stiles, 1990)

Professional Competencies

A. Assess fears of the patient and family in a compassionate, competent, and nonjudgmental manner.

B. Facilitate interdisciplinary consults.

C. Provide for access to spiritual, social, and economic resources.
(Friedman et al., 1999; Reimer et al., 1991; Stiles, 1990)

References

Amenta, M. (1997). Guest editorial. Spiritual care: The heart of palliative nursing. *International Journal of Palliative Nursing, 3,* 1.

Friedman, L., Harrold, J., & Lynne, J. (1999). Care of the dying patient. In M. Beers & R. Berkow (Eds.), *The Merck manual* (17th ed.) (pp. 2509–2516). Whitehouse Station, NJ: Merck Research Laboratories.

Geist, J., & Jefferson, J. (1999). Anxiety disorders. In M. Beers & R. Berkow (Eds.), *The Merck manual* (17th ed.) (pp. 1512–1519).Whitehouse Station, NJ: Merck Research Laboratories.

Kaplan, H., & Sadock, B. (1991). *Synopsis of psychiatry* (6th ed.). Baltimore: Williams & Wilkins.

Reimer, J.C., Davies, B., & Martens, N. (1991). Palliative care: The nurse's role in helping families through the transition of 'fading away.' *Cancer Nursing, 14,* 321–327.

Stiles, M. (1990). The shining stranger: Nurse-family spiritual relationship. *Cancer Nursing, 13,* 235–245.

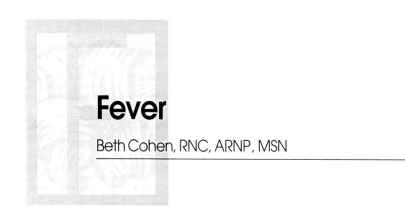

Fever

Beth Cohen, RNC, ARNP, MSN

Definition

Fever refers to an abnormally high body temperature usually occurring in response to pyrogens.

Pathophysiology/Etiology

A temperature of 98.6° Fahrenheit, or 37° Celsius, when taken orally, usually is considered normal or afebrile; however, some individuals may have a body temperature slightly higher or lower than normal. Temperature elevations can occur for reasons independent of illness, such as a very hot environment. Other possible causes include dehydration, medication reaction (drug fever), inflammation, infection, or tumor fevers. Slight elevations in temperature do not bother many patients, whereas others are profoundly bothered by elevations of only 1°–2°. Patients who are actively dying often experience a febrile state (Kirton, Taloffa, & Zwolski, 2000).

Manifestations

- Fatigue
- Skin warmth
- Tachycardia
- Dizziness
- Shortness of breath
- Diaphoresis
- Cold intolerance
- Flushed cheeks
- Headache
- Decreased appetite (anorexia)
- Delirium
- Weakness

- Chills
- Body aches
- Lethargy

Management

A. General measures
  1. Comfort measures
     a) Provide extra blankets if patient is cold or just a thin sheet if warm (Greif & Golden, 1994).
     b) Give a tepid- or lukewarm-water sponge bath, ensuring patient does not experience chills. Do not use alcohol to bathe the patient. Alcohol can cause chills, which will raise the body temperature and can be drying to the skin (Casey, Cohen, & Hughes, 1996; Greif & Golden).
  2. Antipyretic medications ($)
     a) Readily available over the counter or by prescription in oral (pills, capsules, or liquids) and rectal (suppository) forms
     b) Included in this category are acetaminophen (Tylenol®), acetylsalicylic acid (aspirin), and ibuprofen (Motrin®).
     c) The side effects vary with the specific medication ordered and include abdominal discomfort, heartburn, tinnitus, and liver function alterations.
     d) If the patient is on oral pain relievers that combine two or more drugs, including an antipyretic, care must be taken not to exceed the total daily dose of antipyretic medication allowed.
     e) Suppository use is contraindicated in patients with bowel obstruction, diarrhea, or problematic hemorrhoids.
     f) Enteric-coated pills must not be crushed prior to administration (Casey et al.; Greif & Golden; Hodgson & Kizior, 2001; Paganar & Paganar, 1998).
  3. Hydration ($–$$)
     a) Given by mouth, hypodermoclysis, or intravenously
     b) Used to prevent dehydration and electrolyte imbalance
     c) Water at room temperature for a patient who is able to swallow (Casey et al.; Greif & Golden; Hodgson & Kizior).
  4. Antibiotics ($$–$$$)
     a) Chosen if the underlying cause is infection
     b) Choice of medication may be based on sensitivities derived from culture results.
     c) Administration may be oral or intravenous (Casey et al.; Hodgson & Kizior; Kirton et al., 2000).

B. Death is imminent.
  1. Dependent upon patient's and/or family's wishes, attempts to treat the cause of the fever may be abandoned.

2. Comfort measures should continue.
3. If the patient is more comfortable with the use of antipyretics and hydration, they may be continued.

Patient Outcomes

A. Comfort is maintained.

B. Fevers are minimized or eliminated.

Professional Competencies

A. Identify fever and its symptoms.

B. Identify etiology of fever and correct causative factors, when possible.

C. Evaluate the appropriateness and effectiveness of interventions, and modify the treatment plan as needed.

D. Understand the presence of fever as a normal process in the actively dying patient.

References

Casey, K.M., Cohen, F., & Hughes, A. (Eds.). (1996). *ANAC's core curriculum for HIV/AIDS nursing.* Philadelphia: Nurscom.

Greif, J., & Golden, B.A. (1994). *AIDS care at home.* New York: John Wiley & Co.

Hodgson, B., & Kizior, R. (2001). *Saunders nursing drug handbook 2001.* Philadelphia: W.B. Saunders.

Kirton, C.A., Taloffa, D., & Zwolski, K. (Eds.). (2000). *HIV/AIDS nursing handbook.* St. Louis, MO: Mosby.

Paganar, K.D., & Paganar, T.J. (1998). *Mosby's manual of diagnostics and laboratory tests.* St. Louis, MO: Mosby.

Funeral Planning

Jerre Cory, MA, CSW

Definition

Funeral planning is necessary to help lessen the difficulty at the end of life and prevent a crisis situation for family members. Discussing feelings about end-of-life rituals and services eases the grieving process for both the patient and his or her family. The range of planning will vary and depends on one's ability to accept the prognosis. Completing funeral plans in advance reduces financial surprises and answers many questions related to personal wishes.

Specific Issues Related to Palliative Care
Funeral Planning and the Family

Taking care of funeral plans can empower the patient to reduce the feelings of caregiver burden (American Bar Association, 2000). Once this issue is addressed, the patient and his or her family can begin to feel some closure and peacefulness. They then are able to move into productive conversations surrounding other important issues.

Meaning of Funeral Planning to Patient and Family

Finalizing funeral plans does not equate with imminent death. These conversations often are included within advance directives. Talking about and planning for death does not necessarily mean that death is near. More accurately, it promotes the concept that death is a part of life.

Strategies to Facilitate Funeral Planning
Facilitate Communication Surrounding Funeral Plans

Discern the need to encourage funeral planning; this discussion often can be held in combination with discussion of advance directives. The conversations

should include important members of the patient's family. The following questions help target specific needs related to funeral planning.
- Has the patient and family selected a funeral home?
- Has the patient and family discussed disposition of the body (i.e., organ donation, body given to science, earth burial, cremation)?
- Where is the final resting place?
- Is the patient participating in planning the funeral service? Which family members are making the arrangements?
- Are there specific concerns regarding funeral arrangements?

If death is imminent:
- Do not handle death as a crisis (Glass, Cluxton, & Rancour, 2001). This precludes calling emergency numbers such as 911. Instruct the family to call the hospice nurse or physician when death is near or has occurred.
- Provide ongoing reassurance and education to patients and families about what to expect when death is near.
- Prevent a family crisis by reducing fear and confusion at the time of death.

Situational Outcomes

A. Appropriate transition between death setting and transfer to the site for postmortem care

B. Absence of inappropriate use of emergency services at the time of patient's death

Professional Competencies

A. Facilitate funeral planning with patients and their families in a timely and compassionate fashion.

B. Make referrals (e.g., clergy, social worker), as needed, to assist in funeral planning.

References

American Bar Association. (2000). *Five wishes.* Tallahassee, FL: Author.

Glass, E., Cluxton, D., & Rancour, P. (2001). Principles of patient and family assessment. In B. Ferrell & N. Coyle (Eds.), *Textbook of palliative nursing* (pp. 37–50). New York: Oxford University Press.

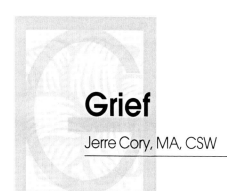

Grief
Jerre Cory, MA, CSW

Definition

Grief is recognized at the onset of loss and mourning (Ersek, 2001). Active grief work often assists patients and their loved ones in recognizing and preparing for impending loss. Grief begins the necessary internal (psychologic and existential) and external (behavioral and social) changes necessary to accommodate loss. Without experiencing acute grief and the learning associated with this phase, mourning will be impeded.

Successful mourning includes the following (Goldman, 2000).

- Coming to grips with the reality of loss by acknowledging and understanding the disease status and letting go of "false" hope that the illness can be reversed
- Reacting to issues of separation from loved ones and finding ways to express and articulate emotional discomfort
- Reviewing memories, thoughts, feelings, hopes, and the stories surrounding loved ones
- Finishing any unfinished business

Specific Issues Related to Palliative Care
Time Limits on Grief

No time limit is set on the grief experience, and it can be activated and reactivated time and time again. Older theories surrounding grief identified a time limit to the grieving process, whereas newer information on grief identifies that grief can recur throughout one's life. How one copes with his or her loss determines whether additional supports are required (Klass, Silverman, & Nickman, 1996).

Types of Grief

The various forms of grief may be misinterpreted. Knowledge of the definitions of grief is important to understand when discerning if the patient and family are moving toward a healthy transition (Ersek, 2001; Goldman, 2000; Klass et al., 1996).

- Anticipatory grief—Often is considered an unconscious process (i.e., learning about a poor prognosis, the anticipation of change that will occur as a result of death).
- Uncomplicated grief—"Normal" grief that is a highly individualized process of loss. The highs and lows of this phase are normal as one adjusts to loss.
- Complicated grief—Ongoing manifestations of prolonged grief that last longer than one year. Individuals are found to repress, deny, avoid any discussion of death, experience intense emotional swings, feel excessively lonely, experience disrupted sleep patterns, lose previous interests, and withdraw socially. Other manifestations include
  - Unusually high death anxiety focusing on self or loved ones
  - Persistent obsessive thoughts and preoccupation with the elements of the loss
  - Inability to experience the various emotional reactions to death
  - Inability to articulate existing feelings and thoughts about the loss
  - Self-destructive behavior
  - Chronic anger
  - Restlessness or overactivity.

Strategies to Promote Healthy Grieving

A. Assess grief reactions and provide appropriate interventions.
  1. Encourage review of positive relationships (in an estranged relationship, note that reconciliation is possible for the griever, even after the patient has died).
  2. Encourage storytelling and looking through photographs.

B. Recognize community resources that may be beneficial for individual needs.
  1. Encourage connections to support groups if this is something that the individual may be interested in doing.
  2. Encourage family members to attend community events that focus on grief and loss, such as seminars, ceremonies, and memorial services.
  3. Become familiar with signs of complicated grief, and provide rapid and appropriate referrals.

Patient or Family Outcomes

A. Individual losses are processed though healthy grieving patterns.

B. Support systems (family members, friends, church groups) help the individual to cope with the loss.

Professional Competencies

A. Identify grief as a normal process, and help support the individual's experience of loss.

B. Assess and evaluate for signs and symptoms of complicated grieving, and make appropriate referrals.

C. Appreciate the interindividuality of grief work.

References

Ersek, M. (2001). The meaning of hope in the dying. In B. Ferrell & N. Coyle (Eds.), *Textbook of palliative nursing* (pp. 339–362). New York: Oxford University Press.

Goldman, L. (2000). *Life and loss.* Philadelphia: Taylor & Francis Publishing.

Klass, D., Silverman, P., & Nickman, S. (1996). *Continuing bonds.* Philadelphia: Taylor & Francis Publishing.

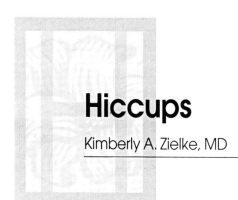

Hiccups

Kimberly A. Zielke, MD

Definition

Hiccups are a pathologic respiratory reflex characterized by a spasm of one or both sides of the diaphragm, resulting in sudden inspiration and closure of the glottis.

Pathophysiology/Etiology

The causes of hiccups are many and varied but can be categorized as one of the following:
- Irritation of the peripheral branches of the phrenic and vagal nerves
- Central nervous system disorders
- Metabolic and drug-induced etiologies
- Infectious disorders
- Psychogenic disturbances
- Idiopathic causes.

Physical examination and laboratory evaluation usually are nondiagnostic. In patients who are dying, gastric distention is probably the most common cause of hiccups (Twycross & Regnarol, 1998).

Manifestations

- Abdominal discomfort
- Mild nausea
- Frustration

Management

A. Death is not imminent.

1. Patients and their families usually have tried a variety of nonpharmacologic maneuvers to control hiccups prior to contacting their healthcare provider. Therefore, if reported, pharmacologic agents usually are prescribed. Peppermint water is used in some centers.
2. Consider a defoaming antiflatulant, like silica-activated simethicone (Maalox-Plus®) ($), before or after meals and at bedtime.
3. If this is ineffective, combine simethicone with a prokinetic drug, such as metoclopramide (Reglan®) ($), 10 mg po 2 or 3 times daily.
4. Other drugs that may be effective include
    a) Baclofen (Lioresal®) ($) 5–20 mg po 2 or 3 times daily
    b) Nifedipine (Procardia®) ($) 10–20 mg po/sl 3 times daily.
5. In resistant cases try
    a) Haloperidol (Haldol®) ($) 2–5 mg po/sq 1 or 2 times daily
    b) Chlorpromazine (Thorazine®) ($) 10–25 mg po 2 or 3 times daily
        (1) This drug almost always works, but adverse effects (e.g., sedation, dry mouth, postural hypotension) are common.
        (2) Titrate to effect, with attention to side effects.
6. Anticonvulsants have been used with varying success. Unless contraindicated, consider
    a) Phenytoin (Dilantin®) ($) 300 mg po/day
    b) Carbamazepine (Tegretol®) ($$) 800 mg po/day (Twycross & Regnarol, 1998).

B. Death is imminent.
    1. Because chlorpromazine ($) is most reliably effective and is available as a suppository, try 50–100 mg pr 2 or 3 times daily.
    2. If the rectal route is not an option, haloperidol ($) may be given subcutaneously 5–10 mg 2 or 3 times daily as needed (Rousseau, 1994).
    3. For patients who are close to death and have persistent, distressing hiccups, a trial of IV or subcutaneous midazolam (Versed®) ($$$) may be necessary (30–120 mg/24 hours) (Wilcock & Twycross, 1996).

Patient Outcomes

A. Minimal to absence of hiccups

B. Minimal to absence of side effects of prescribed medication

Professional Competencies

A. Methods to control/eliminate hiccups are instituted and adjusted to provide optimal control of patient's symptoms.

B. Medications are titrated to obtain optimal benefit with the least side effects.

References

Rousseau, P. (1994). Hiccups in terminal disease. *American Journal of Hospice and Palliative Care, 11,* 7–10.

Twycross, R., & Regnarol, C. (1998). Dysphagia, dyspepsia, and hiccups. In D. Doyle, G.W.C. Hanks, & N. MacDonald (Eds.), *Oxford textbook of palliative medicine* (2nd ed.) (pp. 508–510). New York: Oxford University Press.

Wilcock, A., & Twycross, R. (1996). Case report: Midazolam for intractable hiccups. *Journal of Pain and Symptom Management, 12,* 59–61.

Home or Hospital?

Lynn Borstelmann, RN, MN, CHPN, AOCN®

Decisions regarding the level of care needed at the end of life and the setting in which that care is to be provided must be directed by patient and caregiver goals and expectations and require the input of the entire interdisciplinary team. Patient preferences are priority, but assessment of the individual's medical condition and treatment plan, symptoms, social supports, patient/family financial resources, and available services in the community have to be considered. Many patients state a preference for being cared for at home but may not actually want to die there. Many patients who are hospitalized have a strong desire to return home to die. Patients and family members may have opposite preferences that may change over time.

Specific Issues Related to Palliative Care
Dying at Home

Whether a patient actually dies at home depends on the quality of care and support being provided to both the patient and the caregivers. A key to successful provision of palliative care at home is anticipating possible symptoms and needs before they occur based on expert knowledge of the likely disease progression and the individual patient's history and course. Conditions that increase the likelihood that patients and caregivers will be satisfied with home care and that the death will occur at home include the following (Cantwell et al., 2000; Doyle & Jeffrey, 2000) (see Figure 1).

- Patient and caregiver(s) desire care or death to be at home.
- The quality of pain and symptom control is excellent.
- The level of services provided is adequate for the patient to feel safe/secure and to assist the family members in caring for the patient without undue stress and exhaustion.
- The patient is assured that family members' needs are attended to.
- Patients and families have access to support services 24 hours a day.
- More than one family member or caregiver is in the home to assist.

Figure 1. Advantages and Disadvantages of Home Care

Advantages of Home Care
- Improved quality of life for patients and families: comfort, privacy, familiarity, security, and autonomy
- Reduced focus on illness
- Allows family involvement
- Sustains relationships of family and friends
- Place of memories, happiness, and love
- Confident, relaxed family members
- Familiar care providers

Disadvantages of Home Care
- Small or cramped quarters
- Inadequate facilities
- Inadequate resources
- Fear, anxiety of patient
- Fear, anxiety of family members
- Physical, emotional, and social demands on family members
- Financial loss if family member is out of work to care for patient

---

Note. Based on information from Doyle & Jeffrey, 2000; Stajduhar & Davies, 1998; Woodruff, 1999.

A. Selected criteria for home care (Cantwell et al., 2000; Doyle & Jeffrey, 2000; Stajduhar & Davies, 1998)
   1. Patient and caregiver desire care at home.
   2. Patients with functional limitations and progressive physical deterioration require a willing and able caregiver in the home to provide physical hands-on care and medication administration or to coordinate the efforts of hired staff, family members, or volunteers.
   3. Local healthcare agencies (such as hospice) that can provide comprehensive support in the home should be available, preferably 24 hours a day.
   4. Financial resources or insurance coverage must be sufficient to provide for coverage of needed skilled services from the homecare agency or hospice, equipment, supplies, and medications.
   5. Symptoms must be able to be managed in the home environment.
   6. The home environment must be adequate for the provision of care.
   7. Admission to the hospital or inpatient hospice or palliative care unit can be arranged at short notice if home care breaks down for any reason.

B. Fears about home care (Doyle, 1998)
   1. Worrying about the stress on family members
   2. Fearing readmission to the hospital
   3. Fearing crises
   4. Embarrassing episodes of incontinence, nausea/vomiting, sleeplessness, or confusion
   5. Fear of being excluded from decisions
   6. Fearing impact on children and grandchildren but wanting them close

Dying in a Healthcare Setting

A. Selected criteria for admission to the hospital (see Figure 2)
   1. Difficult to control physical symptoms or suffering, which may include
      a) Intractable breathlessness, nausea/vomiting, or other major uncontrollable symptoms
      b) Fecal incontinence
      c) Hemorrhage
      d) Chronic unproductive cough
      e) Seizures
      f) Malodorous lesions
      g) Cognitive or behavioral issues, especially confusion and agitation
      h) Severe incident/breakthrough pain
   2. Evaluation needed to determine appropriate treatment plan
   3. Recurring crises in the home
   4. Respite for family caregivers
   (Doyle, 1998; Doyle & Jeffrey, 2000)

B. Nursing home alternative
   1. Skilled nursing facilities are an alternative to either home or hospital care, especially if hospice services are available in the nursing home and the patient requires significant amounts of physical care too difficult for family members to provide.

Figure 2. Advantages and Disadvantages of Hospital Care

Advantages of Hospital Care
- Skilled caregivers and technicians
- Specialty medical care
- 24-hour continuous care
- All necessary medications, supplies, and equipment are available.
- Family members may be able to sleep uninterrupted at home if they can stay away from the hospital.

Disadvantages of Hospital Care
- Rigid timetables, regimens, or policies
- Impersonal care
- Loss of control
- Possibility of poor pain control if no palliative care unit/service
- Unnecessary monitoring of vital signs
- Diagnostic and treatment may be of questionable value at this stage of illness.
- Focus on intervention and control of disease rather than comfort
- Social, psychologic, or spiritual needs may be ignored.
- Fragmentation of care
- Decreased involvement of patient and family in care and communication
- Financial cost
- Traveling distance for family, friends
- Patient may not be accepted for admission for terminal care if acute care needs do not exist.

Note. Based on information from Stajduhar & Davies, 1998; Woodruff, 1999.

---

  a) Family members may be more satisfied with care in a facility that has hospice care available (Baer & Hanson, 2000).

  b) In general, however, the nursing home is a less satisfactory alternative to hospital care because of the lack of physician and nursing expertise in palliative care in this setting (Doyle & Jeffrey, 2000).

 2. Inpatient hospice facilities are available in some communities and may be another alternative to nursing home, hospital, or home care.

Strategies to Identify Optimal Place of Death

A. Discuss patient/caregiver preferences for the place of death.

B. Discuss the advantages and disadvantages of the possible places for death to occur.

C. Evaluate the resources available to the patient/caregiver(s) based on their preference for place of death.

D. Provide opportunities for reassessment of preferences as the patient's condition changes.

Patient Outcomes

A. Patient and caregivers will have input into the environment the patient will reside in until death.

B. Patient will be in the environment of choice when possible.

C. Patient's choice of setting will be made based on accurate information and realistic goals and expectations.

Professional Competencies

A. Determine the patient's/caregivers' preferences for location of care.

B. Provide information to patient/caregivers related to options for care and resources.

C. Determine caregiver ability and financial resources to provide care at home.

D. Evaluate psychosocial factors that influence the choice of care setting.

E. Assess adequacy of home environment to support care provision.

F. Provide emotional support to patient and family through active listening, presence, therapeutic use of self and humor, and active development of relationship.

G. Advocate as needed to support patient/caregiver preferences for care setting (i.e., appropriate use of referrals).

References

Baer, W.M., & Hanson, L.C. (2000). Families' perception of the added value of hospice in the nursing home. *Journal of the American Geriatric Society, 48,* 879–882.

Cantwell, P., Turco, S., Brenneis, C., Hanson, J., Neumann, C.M., & Bruera, E. (2000). Predictors of home death in palliative care cancer patients. *Journal of Palliative Care, 16,* 23–28.

Doyle, D. (1998). Domiciliary palliative care. In D. Doyle, G.W.C. Hanks, & N. MacDonald (Eds.), *Oxford textbook of palliative medicine* (2nd ed.) (pp. 957–973). New York: Oxford University Press.

Doyle, D., & Jeffrey, D. (2000). *Palliative care in the home.* New York: Oxford University Press.

Stajduhar, K.I., & Davies, B. (1998). Death at home: Challenges for families and directions for the future. *Journal of Palliative Care, 14,* 8–14.

Woodruff, R. (1999). *Palliative medicine: Symptomatic and supportive care for patients with advanced cancer and AIDS* (3rd ed.). New York: Oxford University Press.

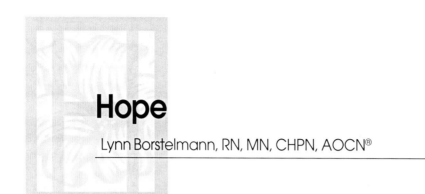

Hope

Lynn Borstelmann, RN, MN, CHPN, AOCN®

Definition

Hope is an essential component of human life. Hope is an inner force that provides direction for the human spirit.

Maintaining a sense of hopefulness and continuing to find meaning in living are the keys to emotional and spiritual health even when life is limited. Hope can be maintained and regenerated through healthy grieving of losses and refocusing on specific goals. People who have lost hope may not desire to continue living. Situations that lead to despair include loss, difficult decisions, uncertainty, or suffering. Pervasive and profound hopelessness is symptomatic of clinical depression. Hopelessness is an independent factor in predicting suicidal thoughts or desire for a hastened death. Maintaining hopefulness and alleviating fears are important for both the patient and caregivers.

Specific Issues Related to Palliative Care
Dimensions of Hope

Hope plays an important role in effective coping and shapes perceptions of quality of life. Research has described dimensions of hope as identified by patients with cancer or advanced illnesses (Ersek, 2001; Nowotny, 1989). These dimensions include
- Confidence in the outcome (treatment, supportive care)
- Ability to relate to others (especially the quality of relationships)
- Possibility of a future (by reframing hope for cure to hope for longer life or hope for comfortable death)
- Spiritual beliefs (relation to a higher being, finding meaning in life)
- Active involvement in achieving and experiencing significant events
- Strength that comes from within (pride, courage, positive outlook, optimism, coping)
- Impacts of physical health, finances, and functional and cognitive abilities.

Threats to Hope

A. Include acute, chronic, and/or terminal illness; cognitive decline; fatigue; and impaired functional status (Ersek, 2001).

B. In advanced illness, these also include the physical and emotional loss of others, poorly controlled pain and other symptoms, physical deterioration, and being treated in a depersonalized manner (Benzein & Saveman, 1998; Herth, 1990).

C. Healthcare professionals who communicate to patients that "nothing more can be done" may generate feelings of hopelessness (Woodruff, 1999).

D. Threats to hope found in family caregivers include isolation from support networks and the practice of religion; concurrent losses, including loss of significant others, health, and income; and an inability to control the patient's symptoms (Ersek, 2001; Herth, 1993).

E. Research has found that caregivers with poor health status, high fatigue, multiple losses, and sleep disturbances are less hopeful.

Hope in Diverse Populations

A. Core concepts and components of hope have been studied across populations varying in health/illness, age, and location of care; however, there is little research that documents ethnic differences.

B. Factors that may affect the multicultural experience or expression of hope include cultural differences in time orientation, value for truth telling, and control.

C. Variations exist in how age affects perceptions of hope (Ersek, 2001).
   1. Younger children are more present-oriented and see adults as being in control.
   2. Older children and their parents have been found to be more hopeful when physical discomforts were well managed.
   3. Children and parents feel cared for when anger can be expressed without judgment, boredom is relieved, and assistance is provided with making and altering plans.
   4. Elderly patients express hope in terms of spiritual well-being, religious beliefs, and concern for loved ones. Threats to hope in the elderly include witnessing hopelessness in others, lack of energy, impaired cognitive function, suffering, and pain experienced by oneself and others.

D. Hopelessness is a symptom of depression and a factor that can predict suicidal thoughts, a desire for hastened death, and an accomplishment of suicide (Breitbart et al., 2000; Chochinov, Wilson, Enns, & Lander, 1998).

E. Depression in the terminally ill is frequently underdiagnosed and undertreated, and symptoms of depression and hopelessness require timely assessment and intervention (Doyle & Jeffrey, 2000).

Strategies to Promote Hope and Prevent Hopelessness

A. Interventions to maintain or support hope and positive energy are integral to the philosophy and practice of palliative care. An interdisciplinary team that provides consistency and continuity of presence and care can support hope.

B. Nursing interventions have been developed by researching cancer and terminally ill patients' own strategies for maintaining hope (Ersek, 2001; Herth, 1990; Nekolaichuk & Bruera, 1998).
   1. Controlling symptoms to satisfy patient/family goals for relief
   2. Providing presence and active listening
   3. Fostering and developing interpersonal connectedness and relationships (family, friends, healthcare professionals)
   4. Maintaining lightheartedness and humor
   5. Identifying, supporting, and reinforcing personal attributes of determination, courage, and serenity
   6. Assisting in the formulation and attainment of specific, achievable goals (refocusing from cure)
   7. Supporting and facilitating engagement with spiritual life
   8. Providing opportunities for life review, focusing on the positive and uplifting
   9. Providing unconditional acceptance of the patient and maintenance of dignity
   10. Balancing support and hopefulness while providing truthful information regarding disease progression and prognosis
   11. Assessing for extreme unrealistic hopes
   12. Utilizing appropriate interdisciplinary team members

C. Interventions specific to family caregivers include the following (Chapman & Pepler, 1998; Ersek, 2001; Herth, 1993).
   1. Facilitating coping
   2. Facilitating grief expression
   3. Encouraging maintenance of social support network
   4. Planning for conservation of caregiver energy
   5. Protecting caregiver physical well-being
   6. Refocusing hope from cure to comfort

Patient Outcomes

A. Realistic hope is maintained.

B. A sense of peacefulness is experienced.

Professional Competencies

A. Use therapeutic communication.

B. Demonstrate appropriate psychosocial assessment skills, especially in identifying potential depression or unhealthy denial.

C. Demonstrate appropriate timing in directing the care focus from cure to comfort.

D. Incorporate counseling skills specific to grief and loss.

E. Recognize the importance of interdisciplinary referrals and teamwork in providing psychosocial and spiritual assessment and care for patients and families.

References

Benzein, E., & Saveman, B.I. (1998). Nurses' perception of hope in patients with cancer: A palliative care perspective. *Cancer Nursing, 21,* 10–16.

Breitbart, W., Rosenfeld, B., Pessin, H., Kaim, M., Funesti-Esch, J., Galietta, M., et al. (2000). Depression, hopelessness, and desire for hastened death in terminally ill patients with cancer. *JAMA, 284,* 2907–2911.

Chapman, K.J., & Pepler, C. (1998). Coping, hope, and anticipatory grief in family members in palliative home care. *Cancer Nursing, 21,* 226–234.

Chochinov, H.M., Wilson, K.G., Enns, M., & Lander, S. (1998). Depression, hopelessness, and suicidal ideation in the terminally ill. *Psychosomatics, 39,* 366–370.

Doyle, D., & Jeffrey, D. (2000). *Palliative care in the home.* New York: Oxford University Press.

Ersek, M. (2001). The meaning of hope in the dying. In B. Ferrell & N. Coyle (Eds.), *Textbook of palliative nursing* (pp. 339–351). New York: Oxford University Press.

Herth, K. (1990). Fostering hope in terminally-ill people. *Journal of Advanced Nursing, 15,* 1250–1259.

Herth, K. (1993). Hope in the family caregiver of terminally ill people. *Journal of Advanced Nursing, 18,* 538–548.

Nekolaichuk, C.L., & Bruera, E. (1998). On the nature of hope in palliative care. *Journal of Palliative Care, 14,* 36–42.

Nowotny, M.L. (1989). Assessment of hope in patients with cancer: Development of an instrument. *Oncology Nursing Forum, 16,* 57–61.

Woodruff, R. (1999). *Palliative medicine: Symptomatic and supportive care for patients with advanced cancer and AIDS* (3rd ed.). New York: Oxford University Press.

Hospice Care

Susanne F. Homant, MBA, PhD(c)

Definition

Hospice is an interdisciplinary model of care for those who have reached the final stages of a terminal illness. Medicare states that hospice services are to be used when two physicians deem the patient has fewer than six months to live (Beresford, 1993; Lattanzi-Licht, Mahoney, & Miller, 1998). Hospice encompasses a multidimensional approach to care by addressing the physical, emotional, psychosocial, and spiritual needs of patients and their families. Medicare mandates that hospice services include bereavement support for families up to one year after the patient's death (Bennahum, 1996).

Specific Issues

A. Hospice care usually is provided in a patient's home—Hospice care initially was given in the patient's home but is now delivered in almost any setting where the patient is located, including, but not limited to, hospice residences, hospitals, nursing homes, homes for the aged, adult foster care homes, and other assisted living settings (Schmoll & Dixon, 1996).

B. Hospice care is interdisciplinary—A team of interdisciplinary professionals develops the plan of care to meet the multiple needs of the patient and family at life's end. The patient and family are considered the center of care, and decisions are based upon their personal goals and realistic expectations. The various disciplines that encompass the core interdisciplinary team include a physician, nurse, social worker, and spiritual care coordinator. Additional members of the interdisciplinary team include nurse aides, physical and occupational therapists, and respite volunteers (Martinez, 1996).

C. Limitations related to hospice care—The knowledge deficit of healthcare providers who fail to refer patients with terminal illnesses other than cancer can interfere with patients' access to hospice services. Initially, hospice care was built upon a malignancy model that included a clear disease progression.

Patients living with advanced illness that does not involve malignancy often are not referred into hospice care. Lack of physician referral earlier in the course of illness is problematic and contributes to very short length of stay in hospice. Physicians and nurses must be knowledgeable about the criteria for admission to hospice service (Kuebler & Berry, 2002).

Strategies to Improve the Use of Hospice Services

A. Identify hospice appropriateness as early as possible.
1. The specialized interdisciplinary team can provide patients and their families with expertise on pain and symptom management and the psychosocial and spiritual issues often confronting patients and their families.
2. Referring patients into this service earlier will prevent fragmented and crisis-oriented care.

B. Empower patients and their families at life's end.
1. Patient- and family-centered care is the locus of the interdisciplinary team's intervention plan.
2. The Medicare hospice benefit requires at least bimonthly interdisciplinary team meetings to discuss issues specific to patients.
3. No single discipline exerts any more or less authority than the other; hospice care is patient and family driven (Lattanzi-Licht et al., 1998; Martinez, 1996).

C. Make full use of insurance reimbursement. Most reimbursement structures ascribe to the capitated Medicare cost/benefit package and will cover the care costs associated with terminal illness, including the cost of
1. Durable medical equipment
2. Interdisciplinary services
3. Medical supplies
4. Pharmaceuticals
5. Ancillary services.

D. Offer the most appropriate level of care; hospice offers four levels.
1. Routine care: The patient receives routine care while remaining at home with the support of the interdisciplinary team.
2. Continuous care: Prolonged skilled nursing services are provided in the patient's home if the patient or his or her family is experiencing unrelieved symptoms.
3. Inpatient care
   a) This level of care is provided in a facility (e.g., hospital, hospice residence, nursing home) to provide complex symptom management that cannot be given in the home.
   b) This level of care can only be given for a limited period of time.
4. Respite care

a) Respite care can be provided in either a facility or the patient's home and is designed to give caregivers a rest from the physical, emotional, and spiritual demands of patient care.

b) Respite care is limited to five days and nights at a time (Lattanzi-Licht et al., 1998).

Patient Outcomes

A. Admission to hospice services is timely.

B. Patient receives continuity of care between primary provider and supportive services.

C. Patient remains pain- and symptom-free until death.

D. Family members receive supportive services and bereavement care.

Professional Competencies

A. Identify prognostic indicators of advanced illness that warrant a referral to hospice care.

B. Identify one's own thoughts and feelings about death and dying when providing care for the terminally ill.

C. Educate patients and families regarding the purpose and benefits of hospice care (Beresford, 1993; Zeefe, 1996).

References

Bennahum, D. (1996). The historical development of hospice and palliative care. In D. Sheehan & W. Forman (Eds.), *Hospice and palliative care: Concepts and practice* (pp. 1–11). Boston: Jones and Bartlett.

Beresford, L. (1993). *The hospice handbook.* Boston: Little, Brown & Co.

Kuebler, K., & Berry, P. (2002). End-of-life care. In K. Kuebler, P. Berry, & D. Heidrich (Eds.), *End-of-life care: Clinical practice guidelines for advanced practice nursing* (pp. 23–37). Philadelphia: W.B. Saunders.

Lattanzi-Licht, M., Mahoney, J., & Miller, G. (1998). *The hospice choice.* New York: Simon & Schuster.

Martinez, J. (1996). The interdisciplinary team. In D. Sheehan & W. Forman (Eds.), *Hospice and palliative care: Concepts and practice* (pp. 21–31). Boston: Jones and Bartlett.

Schmoll, B., & Dixon, C. (1996). Hospice care settings. In D. Sheehan & W. Forman (Eds.), *Hospice and palliative care: Concepts and practice* (pp. 51–61). Boston: Jones and Bartlett.

Zeefe, L. (1996). Death education: Teaching staff, patients, and families about the dying process. In D. Sheehan & W. Forman (Eds.), *Hospice and palliative care: Concepts and practice* (pp. 107–115). Boston: Jones and Bartlett.

Infection

Peg Esper, MSN, RN, CS, AOCN®

Definition

Infection is the invasion of the body by foreign organisms that disrupt host homeostasis.

Pathophysiology/Etiology

Patients with advanced illnesses are at heightened risk for infection. This increased risk is a result of a number of factors, including, but not limited to, decreased nutrition status, depressed immune function secondary to past treatment, disease progression, steroid use, immobility leading to skin breakdown, and indwelling catheters (Kemp, 1999).

Manifestations

Manifestations are dependent on the site of infection and include the following.
- Fever
- Pain
- Purulent discharge
- Mouth sores
- Erythema
- Localized warmth
- Malodorous drainage
- Cough
- Dyspnea
- Hematuria
- Tachycardia
- Tachypnea
- Rigors
- Edema

Management

The priority of management is to try and prevent infection whenever possible. Measures to prevent infection include
- Avoiding contact with known pathogens or carriers
- Meticulous skin or wound care
- Optimal activity
- Regular changing of indwelling catheters
- Antibiotic prophylaxis when appropriate
- Regular oral hygiene.

A. Death is not imminent: Although infection frequently can be the cause of death for individuals with advanced illnesses, attempts should be made to treat infections after they are identified.
   1. General measures
      a) Antipyretic administration
      b) Analgesics as indicated
   2. Treatments for suspected respiratory tract infection
      a) Broad-spectrum antibiotics ($)—trimethoprim and sulfamethoxazole (Bactrim®), ampicillin (Amoxil®), azithromycin (Zithromax®) (Regnard & Tempest, 1998)
      b) Consider the use of an antibiotic in liquid form for patients with dysphagia.
      c) Suspected *Pneumocystis carinii* should be treated with co-trimoxazole (Cotrim®) 60 mg/kg po/IV q 12 hours x 2 weeks (Regnard & Tempest).
   3. Treatment for urinary tract infection (UTI)
      a) Encourage increased fluids, especially those that increase urine acidity.
      b) Antibiotics ($–$$)—UTIs often can be treated with a short course of antibiotics, but recurrence is common and maintenance dosing may be required. Typical antibiotic treatments for UTI include ampicillin (Amoxil®), ciprofloxacin (Cipro®), trimethoprim and sulfamethoxazole, nitrofurantoin (Macrodantin®) (maintenance) (Berry, 1999; Kemp, 1999).
      c) Change indwelling urinary catheters on a regular basis.
      d) Phenazopyridine (Pyridium®) ($)100–200 mg po qid for comfort (Kemp)
      e) Review procedure being used for intermittent self-catheterization.
   4. Fungal/yeast infections
      a) Keep site clean and dry if outside of oral cavity.
      b) Topical/oral antifungal agents ($–$$)—For oral candidiasis, topical antifungals require a long mucosal contact time to be effective, meaning frequent dosing. Oral antifungals, such as fluconazole (Diflucan®), may be more effective (Ventafridda, Ripamonte, Sbanotto, & DeConno, 1998).
      c) Monitor for recurrence.

5. Catheter infections
   a) Change catheters regularly (following product guidelines/policy and procedure guidelines) ($–$$$), including percutaneous nephrostomy tubes and IV catheters (Norman, 1998).
   b) Antibiotic administration ($–$$$)—Specific antibiotic depends on type of organism involved.
   c) Regular cleansing around the catheter insertion site
6. Wound infections (See Skin Lesions.)

B. Death is imminent.
1. When death is anticipated to be within a matter of days, the use of antibiotics may not be appropriate.
2. In these situations, comfort is the priority and the following measures should be instituted.
   a) Management of fever/chills (Rhiner & Slatkin, 2001)
   b) Management of dyspnea and cough (use of oxygen, opiates) (See Cough and Dyspnea sections.)
   c) Management of drainage/odor from infection, wounds, or catheter sites (See Skin Lesions.)
   d) Analgesic support as needed (See Pain.)

Patient Outcomes

A. Patients are aware of signs and symptoms related to infection that need to be reported to their healthcare provider.

B. Infection is treated when possible.

C. When death is imminent, comfort is maintained.

Professional Competencies

A. Identify patient risk factors for various types of infections.

B. Establish a plan for prevention of infection when possible.

C. Determine the best method to manage infection based on patient condition, type of infection, and resources available.

D. Identify comfort measures to be instituted when infection is not treatable and death is imminent.

E. Evaluate effectiveness of plan and modify as appropriate.

References

Berry, D. (1999). Bladder disturbances. In C. Yarbro, M. Frogge, & M. Goodman (Eds.), *Cancer symptom management* (pp. 489–498). Boston: Jones and Bartlett.

Kemp, C. (1999). *Terminal illness* (2nd ed.). Philadelphia: J.B. Lippincott.

Norman, R.W. (1998). Genitourinary disorders. In D. Doyle, G.W.C. Hanks, & N. MacDonald (Eds.), *Oxford textbook of palliative medicine* (2nd ed.) (pp. 667–676). New York: Oxford University Press.

Regnard, C., & Tempest, S. (1998). *A guide to symptom relief in advanced disease* (4th ed.). Hale, England: Hochland & Hochland.

Rhiner, M., & Slatkin, N. (2001). Pruritus, fever and sweats. In B. Ferrell & N. Coyle (Eds.), *Textbook of palliative nursing* (pp. 245–260). New York: Oxford University Press.

Ventafridda, V., Ripamonte, C., Sbanotto, A., & DeConno, F. (1998). Mouth care. In D. Doyle, G.W.C. Hanks, & N. MacDonald (Eds.), *Oxford textbook of palliative medicine* (2nd ed.) (pp. 691–707). New York: Oxford University Press.

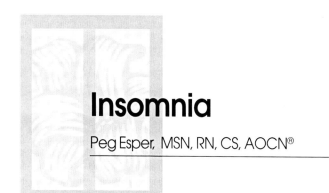

Insomnia

Peg Esper, MSN, RN, CS, AOCN®

Definition

Insomnia is the inability to sleep when desired.

Pathophysiology/Etiology

Insomnia can have profound effects on both the patient and his or her caregiver. The inability to sleep may be related to physiologic as well as psychologic factors. Uncontrolled symptoms—such as pain, nausea, pruritus, cough, xerostomia, and dyspnea—are frequently associated with insomnia. In addition, fear, anxiety, agitation, depression, and confusion are also possible contributing factors related to the inability to sleep. Certain medications (e.g., psychostimulants, steroids) can also lead to insomnia. The exact physiologic mechanism involved is dependent on the etiology of the insomnia. Patients are likely to experience one or many of the stressors that interfere with sleep at some point while receiving palliative care. These can include fear of not waking up, fear of being alone at night, and "mind wandering" when other stimuli is at a minimum (Sateia & Silberfarb, 1998). Patients may be physically separated from their usual "sleepmate" or in a bed that is not their own (Yellen & Dyonzak, 1999).

Manifestations

- Tossing and turning rather than sleeping
- Awakening after only sleeping a short time
- Awakening in the early morning
- Fatigue
- Decreased cognition
- Confusion
- Delirium
- Agitation

- Fear of the unknown
- Distressing dreams

Management

A. Evaluate the patient's sleep patterns.
   1. Does the patient sleep during the day?
   2. Does the patient fall asleep but wake up easily?
   3. Is the patient unable to fall asleep?
   4. The number of hours generally slept each night
   5. Current use of any sleep aids
   6. History of sleeping problems
   7. Current setting for sleep (e.g., room, bed, who is with the patient)

B. Evaluate current medication profile for agents that may interfere with sleep, and modify as feasible.

C. Institute general measures to help promote sleep (Kemp, 1999).
   1. Limit daytime naps when possible.
   2. Avoid intake of stimulant foods/beverages near bedtime.
   3. Provide an environment conducive to sleep (e.g., amount of light, level of sound) based on patient preference.
   4. Institute comfort measures (e.g., control any pain, egg-crate mattress for bed, extra pillows, sheepskin).
   5. Establish a bedtime routine.

D. Institute measures to deal with the physical and psychologic issues contributing to insomnia (Kemp, 1999; Yellen & Dyonzak, 1999).
   1. Counsel as appropriate to identify and address fears surrounding death.
   2. Use low-level lighting.
   3. Provide means for patient to call for assistance quickly (e.g., bell, intercom system, sitters).
   4. Use music or other audio distractors (e.g., relaxation tapes).
   5. Aromatherapy
   6. Hypnosis
   7. Guided imagery
   8. Massage
   9. Encourage prayer and/or meditation.

E. Pharmacologic agents: These may be used singly or in combination to decrease insomnia (Kemp, 1999; Sateia & Silberfarb, 1998; Yellen & Dyonzak, 1999).
   1. Antianxiety agents ($–$$) (See Anxiety.)
   2. Hypnotics ($–$$)—zolpidem (Ambien®), triazolam (Halcion®), temazepam (Restoril®)
   3. Antidepressants ($–$$) (See Depression.)

F. Nonprescription agents (Yellen & Dyonzak, 1999)
   1. Melatonin ($–$$)—Data remain questionable, but some benefit is noted in the elderly.
   2. Valerian root extract ($–$$)—Care must be taken, as preparations are not uniformly controlled.

G. Treatment of additional conditions contributing to insomnia (e.g., xerostomia)

Patient Outcomes

A. Satisfactory periods of sustained sleep are attained.

B. Rest is adequate to allow participation in meaningful activities.

Professional Competencies

A. Identify individual physical and psychologic factors that contribute to insomnia.

B. Institute measures to enhance the patient's sleep.

C. Evaluate effectiveness of specific interventions, and modify the plan as appropriate.

Measurement Tools

A. Sleep diary

B. Caregiver's observations

References

Kemp, C. (1999). *Terminal illness* (2nd ed.). Philadelphia: J.B. Lippincott.

Sateia, M., & Silberfarb, P. (1998). Sleep. In D. Doyle, G.W.C. Hanks, & N. MacDonald (Eds.), *Oxford textbook of palliative medicine* (2nd ed.) (pp. 751–767). New York: Oxford University Press.

Yellen, S., & Dyonzak, J. (1999). Sleep disturbances. In C. Yarbro, M. Frogge, & M. Goodman (Eds.), *Cancer symptom management* (pp. 161–173). Boston: Jones and Bartlett.

Insurance

Lynn Borstelmann, RN, MN, CHPN, AOCN®

The Medicare hospice benefit is the most significant source of patient coverage and agency reimbursement available to cover the cost of end-of-life care. The Medicaid hospice benefit is very similar and implemented in most states. Commercial insurance coverage for the needs of palliative care patients varies a great deal based on plan benefits. Providers need to be aware of the limits of patient insurance coverage and financial resources to negotiate the best possible services and coverage for palliative care patients and their families.

Specific Issues Related to Palliative Care
Coverage for Hospice Care
The Medicare hospice benefit is a per diem benefit for terminally ill patients who have a prognosis of six months or fewer. The benefit covers four levels of care with prescribed criteria for each level: routine home care, continuous care, general inpatient care, and respite care. The program pays 100% of intermittent nursing, social work, physician services, counseling/pastoral services, home-health aide, physical/occupational therapy, durable medical equipment and supplies, and other therapies, as needed, related to the terminal illness (Emanuel, von Gunten, & Ferris, 1999).

Advantages of the Medicare hospice benefit include
- Coverage of medications related to the terminal illness (Medicare does not otherwise cover medications for outpatients.)
- Interdisciplinary care, including psychosocial and spiritual care
- Hospitalization, if needed, for medication adjustment, observation, stabilization, psychosocial monitoring, or if a family becomes unwilling to provide care at home
- Bereavement follow-up.

Hospices are permitted to charge a small co-pay for medicines and respite care, although most do not.

Disadvantages include
- Requirement for physician certification in cases in which prognosis is for fewer than six months

- Patient acceptance of care
- Discontinuity in relationships with healthcare providers in the transition from home health to hospice care
- Potential limits on patient access to more invasive or expensive treatment modalities that are incompatible with the philosophy of hospice care or the low per diem rate structure (Field & Cassel, 1997).

Patients living in a nursing home may access their Medicare hospice benefit to obtain hospice services if another source of payment/reimbursement is allowed for the nursing home room and board fees. Not all states have exercised the option to include hospice as a covered Medicaid service. For those that have, the program usually is governed by the same Centers for Medicare and Medicaid Services guidelines as the Medicare benefit. Commercial insurance coverage for hospice care varies widely, with many insurance plans providing services similar to those of the Medicare hospice model (Egan & Labyak, 2001), some providing services within a traditional home health model, and some providing no coverage at all. An estimated 80% of large and medium-sized employers offer some type of hospice coverage (Field & Cassel, 1997). Some states require that commercial insurers include hospice care as a covered benefit.

Coverage for Home Care

Medicare and Medicaid home health benefits also can cover the cost of palliative care at home within the limits of regulatory guidelines for these programs. Medicare home health coverage is restricted to patients who meet the criteria for being homebound and are receiving medically necessary, skilled services, part-time or intermittent, from the disciplines of nursing, physical therapy, or speech therapy (Milone-Nuzzo & McCorkle, 2001). Coverage of home health aides also is included, and durable medical equipment is covered separately at 80%. Limited coverage is available for social work services, and no coverage is given for pastoral or bereavement care. A physician must sign and oversee the treatment plan (Milone-Nuzzo & McCorkle). A prospective payment system for Medicare home health benefits was mandated by the Balanced Budget Act of 1997 and was implemented in October 2000. Medicare no longer reimburses agencies by the visit, and home health agencies now must provide medically necessary supplies (except for durable medical equipment) along with skilled services. The incentives for keeping patients with costly care in the program for longer periods of time is changing as a result of the revised reimbursement structure. Commercial insurance coverage for palliative care at home also may be very limited—a fixed number of skilled nursing visits (with no coverage for interdisciplinary care or bereavement follow-up) may be covered. Some patients with extended illnesses may reach the maximum lifetime benefit and may lose coverage (Milone-Nuzzo & McCorkle). Medications usually are covered with plans that include prescription benefits.

Coverage for Inpatient Care and Palliative Care Services

Inpatient palliative care traditionally is provided and reimbursed through general inpatient care insurance coverage, whether Medicare, Medicaid, or commercial insurance. Patients may be discharged prematurely because the perception is that terminal care does not require acute care admission. Very few commercial insurance plans provide specific palliative care benefits, whether for home care, long-term care, or inpatient hospital care. For palliative services that are provided in traditional hospitals, patients usually must meet criteria for acute care, and this poses problems when patients require hospitalization for caregiving issues or lack of homecare support. The hospital care coordinator may be able to negotiate reimbursement with commercial insurers for the level of care that the patient requires in the inpatient setting or may encourage transfer of the patient to an alternative care setting.

Coverage for Long-Term Care

Insurance coverage for long-term care also is limited. Medicare skilled nursing facility (SNF) coverage is not intended to cover the costs of chronic, long-term care (Zerzan, Stearns, & Hanson, 2000). Patients experiencing terminal illness may receive some time-limited coverage through the skilled nursing benefit, as long as they meet the resource utilization group criteria and a facility is willing to admit them. The maximum number of days covered is 100 per episode of illness, and there is a $97 copay per day for days 21–100. The patient must have a three-day qualifying stay in an acute-care hospital. Medicare covers either hospice care or care in a nursing home, not both. Patients with Medicare and Medicaid coverage may receive hospice care by Medicare, whereas Medicaid covers nursing home room and board (Zerzan et al.) Medicaid covers short-term rehabilitation and long-term care in a nursing home if criteria for income or disability are met. Medicaid will cover both hospice care and nursing home care in states with a Medicaid hospice benefit (Zerzan et al.). Frail elderly patients eligible for Medicare and Medicaid may be enrolled in a Program of All-Inclusive Care of the Elderly that provides comprehensive medical and social services in a daycare center, with the goal of integrating acute-care and long-term care services and preventing admission to a nursing home. Patients with traditional commercial insurance or managed-care benefits may or may not have long-term care coverage, usually for a specific number of days or an episode of illness.

Limits to Coverage

The best clinical treatment and supportive care plans for patients and families may or may not be supported by the patient's insurance plan and financial resources. Some institutions and settings of care may have a wider latitude to provide services to patients who are without adequate insurance; other institutions provide services through alternative means of funding and support (e.g., grants, charitable fundraising, Hill-Burton Act). Institutions with inpatient palliative care or hospice units may have specially negotiated rates with insurers for this level of care. Patients who are ill for long periods of time may lose access to employer-sponsored health insurance and wind up without coverage (Field & Cassel, 1997).

No insurers other than Medicaid will consider payment for a custodial level of care. This puts a burden on families to provide basic care and assistance for patients at home, whether the patient's overall care plan is being supervised by a certified hospice or homecare agency. Families experience a significant financial impact as a result of lack of insurance when a loved one has a terminal illness. They are responsible for out-of-pocket medical expenses not covered by insurance, medications and supplies, paid caregiving assistance, and the need to take unpaid time from work (Field & Cassel, 1997).

Other Sources of Coverage

Community agencies and nonprofit organizations—such as the American Cancer Society, Leukemia and Lymphoma Society of America, and other disease-specific or community-based programs—may provide assistance to patients with limited means.

Medications may be obtained for patients with limited financial means through pharmaceutical assistance programs (refer to Resources, later in this section).

Some patients may be able to take advantage of companies offering viatical settlements by selling life insurance policies to provide needed financial resources at the end of life. Companies usually pay 60%–80% of the face value of the policy and require medical record documentation and certification of the chronic or terminal illness by a physician.

Strategies for Handling Insurance Issues

A. Always check patients' health insurance coverage and benefits, and include patients and families in decision making regarding care needs, options, and costs of care.

B. Encourage referral to hospice as early as the plan of care and patient acceptance allow so patients may experience the full benefit of hospice coverage.

C. Develop individualized patient care plans that maximize patient insurance coverage and financial resources to meet patients' needs for end-of-life care.

D. Develop relationships with community agencies to maximize the consideration for the needs of individual patients and patient populations that are served.

E. Develop relationships with commercial insurance and managed care case managers to advocate for the needs of individual patients and families and population groups.

Professional Competencies

A. Incorporate knowledge of Medicare and Medicaid coverage for hospice care, home care, and SNF care in the plan of care.

B. Demonstrate knowledge of various levels of care and care settings available in the community, criteria for admission, and costs of care.

C. Use knowledge of community resources for palliative and hospice care.

D. Incorporate community agency and pharmaceutical manufacturer assistance programs for medications, supplies, transportation, and other needs when necessary.

E. Use skills in client advocacy to negotiate with payors to meet patients' needs.

Resources

A. National Viatical Association—800-741-9465; www.nationalviatical.org/choosing.html

B. Information about drug assistance programs—Pharmaceutical Research and Manufacturers Association of America provides a directory of prescription drug assistance programs: 202-835-3400; www.phrma.org/searchcures/dpdpap/. Other information about prescription drug assistance programs: www .rxhope.com/. Medicare Web site on prescription drug assistance programs: www.medicare.gov/Prescription/Home.asp.

C. Information for Medicare beneficiaries: www.medicare.gov

D. American Association of Health Plans primary trade association for managed care plans—www.aahp.org/AAHP/index.cfm

E. Health Insurance Association of America (primary trade association for health insurers—www.hiaa.org

References

Egan, K.A., & Labyak, M.J. (2001). Hospice care: A model for quality end-of-life care. In B. Ferrell & N. Coyle (Eds.), *Textbook of palliative nursing,* (pp. 7–26). New York: Oxford University Press.

Emanuel, L.L., von Gunten, C.F., & Ferris, F.D. (1999). *The education for physicians on end-of-life care (EPEC) curriculum.* Princeton, NJ: The Robert Wood Johnson Foundation.

Field, M.J., & Cassel, C.K. (Eds.). (1997). Financial and economic issues in end-of-life care. In *Approaching death: Improving care at the end of life* (pp. 154–187). Washington, DC: Institute of Medicine, National Academy Press.

Milone-Nuzzo, P., & McCorkle, R. (2001). Home care. In B. Ferrell & N. Coyle (Eds.), *Textbook of palliative nursing* (pp. 543–555). New York: Oxford University Press.

Zerzan, J., Stearns, S., & Hanson, L. (2000). Access to palliative care and hospice in nursing homes. *JAMA, 284,* 2489–2494.

Isolation

Rev. James M. Deshotels, SJ, APRN

Definition

Isolation is a major risk of end-stage disease, when a person is separated from normal activities of daily life, family, friends, former colleagues, and social involvements. The most likely initial causes of isolation are logistical—termination of employment or confinement to home, hospital, or extended care facility. When family, friends, and acquaintances visit, the patient may be too fatigued to receive company. They eventually become too weak to travel to doctors appointments. Patients with advanced illness feel isolated by their dependent role and the losses associated in the dying process, despite the attention of family and loved ones (Institute of Medicine, 1997; Peralta, 2001; Singer, Martin, & Kelner, 1999).

Specific Issues Related to Palliative Care

Holistic Approach to Care

One of the major contributions of hospice care has been involving the family in the care of their dying loved ones. This holistic approach is a significant factor in reducing the sense of isolation, but issues of isolation may be present even from the family and significant others. Family members need reassurance and guidance because they often feel increasingly incompetent and impotent to deal with dying. This may lead to tension as loved ones try to stay involved in the life and care of the dying person. Family caregivers may become overaggressive with efforts like feeding because of their own anxiety, but the tension itself can lead to exploration and reduction of the anxiety. The end result is greater comfort, including psychosocial and spiritual comfort, for both patient and family.

Abandonment

Patients need and want the assurance that family members and healthcare providers will remain with them and not abandon them as they face death, reassuring them they will not die alone or in pain.

Avoiding Doing Things to Prolong Life Out of the Caregivers' Need to Do Something

During this stage of the patient's care, it becomes far less important to perform certain tasks than to be physically *available.* In today's healthcare climate, providers and families will find their skills and patience tested by social and economic disparities. Effective palliative and terminal care will often include complex case management and access to resources beyond the traditional constraints of predictable and reliable medical care systems. However, the hospice care system is dedicated to integrating and providing these needed resources.

Unfinished Business

Isolation from family and significant others may result from unfinished business or a need for reconciliation and forgiveness. Impending death may be the impetus for such reconciliation—for putting affairs in order and expressing love previously left unspoken. The interdisciplinary team may be the first to recognize and acknowledge the existence of such issues and can facilitate communication among the patient and significant others (Rakel & Storey, 1993; Singer et al., 1999; Stiles, 1990).

Strategies to Prevent Isolation

A. Interventions to diminish isolation may range from the technological to the spiritual: Adequate telephone or computer access may be as important to a patient or family as medications and supplies. (See section on spirituality.)

B. Management guidelines (Peralta, 2001; Singer et al., 1999; Stiles, 1990)
   1. Provide opportunities for patients and families to talk about the losses they have already experienced, are currently experiencing, and those they anticipate.
   2. Acknowledge that patients and significant others will vary in their ability to assimilate the changes and that a range of reactions and coping strategies is normal.
   3. Consider ways to help the patient to be as independent as possible.
   4. Consider ways that the patient can remain involved with family life (prevent social death).
   5. Help to sort out family members' expectations with regard to the dying member, each other, and themselves.
   6. Legitimize respite time, and help patients and family members incorporate it from the outset.
   7. Help patients and family members to understand the dynamics of the situation that contribute to their complex and ambivalent feelings.
   8. Use community resources to support the family when their resources are insufficient.
   9. Appreciate that helping will not always entail finding an answer or a specific solution.

10. Normalize the transition, and help patients and their families understand the dynamics associated with the paradoxes they face (keeping on living while preparing for death).
11. Provide a sounding board for people as they try to sort out their thoughts and feelings.
12. Validate and normalize feelings.
13. Help people explore their options.
14. Be aware of your own comfort level in dealing with situations that are paradoxical and arouse ambivalent feelings.
15. Do not force people to talk about difficult topics, but appraise whether the hesitation comes from within you or the family.
16. Do not focus solely on death and dying; focus also on life and living.
17. Encourage life review, and recognize that this may include regrets and pain as well as pleasant memories.
18. Help patients and families to include children in the process rather exclude them.
19. Affirm patients and families for their ability to manage and create goodness amid tragedy.

Patient Outcomes

A. Communicates feelings of isolation

B. Able to overcome feelings of isolation
(Singer et al., 1999; Stiles, 1990)

Professional Competencies

A. Demonstrate therapeutic listening skills.

B. Facilitate communication between the patient and loved ones.

C. Implement a variety of strategies to resolve patient's/family's feelings of isolation, and modify the plan as appropriate.
(Institute of Medicine, 1997; Peralta, 2001; Rakel & Storey, 1993; Singer et al., 1999; Stiles, 1990)

References

Institute of Medicine. (1997). *Approaching death: Improving care at the end of life.* Washington, DC: National Academy Press.

Peralta, A. (2001, February 15). *Outline and handouts for home health conference call.* St. Louis, MO: Ascension Health.

Rakel, R.E., & Storey, P. (1993). Care of the dying patient. In R.E. Rakel (Ed.), *Essentials of family practice* (pp. 68–81). Philadelphia: W.B. Saunders.

Singer, P.A., Martin, D.K., & Kelner, M. (1999). Quality end-of-life care: Patients' perspectives. *JAMA, 281,* 163–168.

Stiles, M. (1990). The shining stranger: Nurse-family spiritual relationship. *Cancer Nursing, 13,* 235–245.

Legal Issues in Pain Management

Martin Perz, JD

A new legal threshold has been established in relation to a minimum standard of care for the management of patients in pain. This is largely because of a number of events at the national level, including implementation of "pain as the fifth vital sign," by the Veterans Administration Hospitals, the advent of the Joint Commission on Accreditation of Healthcare Organizations (JCAHO) standards for appropriate evaluation and treatment of pain, and the increasing visibility of judgments that have emanated from the inadequate treatment of pain (Joranson & Gilson, 2001; Rich, 2000).

Specific Issues Related to Palliative Care

Healthcare providers have historically pondered the legal consequences of administering opiates in substantial quantities, given the regulatory issues that surround this practice of medicine. Although the consequences to the culpable party can be dire (specifically, licensure restrictions and, in worst-case scenarios, criminal charges), the evidence that this issue routinely surfaces is scant (Joranson & Gilson, 2001). Conversely, many commentators have asserted that the fear of this issue, be it grounded in fact or in urban legend, suppresses the adequate prescribing of opiates for those suffering with malignant pain ("Jury Awards," 1995). The resultant overall effect is that patients suffer needlessly in the name of an excess caution that stems from fear (Rich, 2000). A more complete understanding of the laws governing the prescribing and use of opiates for the legitimate treatment of pain is crucial if this barrier is to be overcome. Fear related to prescribing of analgesics leads to numerous problems.

- Unnecessary patient suffering
- Promulgation of opiate phobia
- Diminished end-stage quality of life for patient and family
- Inadequate amounts of opiates delivered to patient
- Regulatory scrutiny for undertreatment of pain
- Legal judgments

Spheres of Jurisdiction
Drug Enforcement Administration

The Drug Enforcement Administration (DEA) controls the distribution of all scheduled medications under the aegis of the Controlled Substances Act (CSA). The CSA is specifically concerned with diversion issues that result in the illegal sale and subsequent use of opiates for recreational purposes. The DEA does not control the practice of medicine; however, it has the authority to strip DEA licenses and to process criminal charges against caregivers who have been involved in the targeted activities.

A. Governed by the CSA, 21 USC 822, the mission of the DEA is to prevent the diversion of scheduled medications into illicit areas, not to second-guess physicians or critique new therapies (DEA, 1970).

B. DEA is responsible for the registration of professionals who may prescribe controlled substances. No caregiver is permitted to prescribe scheduled medications without a DEA license (Federation of State Medical Boards, 1998).

C. The standard for appraisal by DEA when considering the use of scheduled medications is "utilization of medications for legitimate medical purposes in the usual course of professional practice" (DEA, 1970). DEA does not set these standards for the usual course of practice; rather, individual state boards of medicine set these standards (Joranson & Gilson, 2001).

D. DEA investigations are triggered by egregious behavior, including, but not limited to, the following:
    1. Questionable amounts of opiates for unusual reasons (e.g., a podiatrist receives 500 Percocets per month from a mail-order pharmacy).
    2. Criminal distribution, as determined by street purchases by undercover agents. Specifically, purchases are made from a known dealer on an ongoing basis, many of which have been prescribed by the same physician.
    3. Unusual amounts of self-prescribing wherein a professional is prescribing opiates for himself or herself or for employees and family members. An absolute investigational trigger is the picking up of scheduled medications by a physician, ostensibly for a patient or employee who is "unable" to pick them up for himself or herself.
    4. The prescribing of opiates to maintain or detoxify an addict. *Note:* If addiction occurs as an outgrowth of an acceptable treatment protocol for the treatment of intractable or malignant pain, this is not a DEA issue; however, no one is permitted to maintain or detoxify an addict unless he or she represents a licensed treatment facility for that purpose. (For these purposes, the CSA defines *addict* as a person who "habitually uses any narcotic drug so as to endanger the public morals, health, and safety or who is so far addicted to the use of narcotic drugs as to have lost power of self-control with reference to his addiction" (DEA, 1970).

5. Wholesalers and mail-order pharmacies are required to report, on a quarterly basis, unusual orders for scheduled medications; however:
   a) Large amounts of Class II (CII) regulated medications ordered by hospices are not unusual.
   b) It is expected that those who treat the terminally ill will prescribe large amounts of opiates.
   c) Caregivers are expected to take adequate precautions with their prescriptions and prescription pads and to be diligent in preventing unauthorized use of the same.

E. Almost 100% of DEA investigations involve out-of-hospital practice or, more specifically, the practice of medicine from a clinic or private office.

F. Many investigations do not involve illegal practices but poor judgment on the part of the caregiver, such as:
   1. Lack of diagnostic documentation for long-term prescribing of unusual amounts of opiates
   2. Lack of agreements that allow a single patient to see multiple physicians and receive medications from more than one source
   3. Failure to exercise due care with prescriptions that are stolen or otherwise used by unauthorized parties (e.g., employees, family members, patients).

G. End points
   1. Communication with the DEA always is an option if and when a caregiver has reservations about a given patient.
   2. Professionals are almost always given the benefit of informal or administrative contact, unless extreme evidence of illicit/illegal behavior is uncovered.
   3. A visit from a DEA agent is as likely as a lightning strike.

State Medical Boards

State medical boards control the practice of medicine within their stated jurisdictions. The state boards have the power to assess individual practices of medicine and to weigh the same against the prevailing standards, as they are deemed to exist within the given sphere of practice. State boards have the power to strip licenses to practice within a given jurisdiction but lack the criminal prosecutorial authority of the DEA. State medical boards do, however, work in tandem with the DEA when alerted by DEA agents of suspicious behavior.

A. Medical practice is not regulated by the CSA. The states, not the federal government, have the authority to regulate medical practice. This authority is founded in state constitutions, wherein the states are empowered to draft laws to protect the general health and welfare of their citizenry. The CSA was not intended to supersede the authority of the states in this matter and provides no authority for the DEA to regulate medical decisions.

B. State medical boards administer medical practice laws and have the responsibility of protecting the public health from substandard, incompetent, and unlawful practices. These boards determine what constitutes unprofessional conduct and have the authority to grant, suspend, deny, limit, or revoke a license to practice medicine.

C. The state boards perform investigations into inappropriate practices. These may or may not be prompt, may be dropped because of insufficient evidence, or may proceed to disciplinary action, which may range from a warning, to education, to a limitation or removal of prescribing privilege or the professional license. The state courts may review these actions (Joranson & Gilson, 2001).

D. State medical boards govern the practice of opiate treatment by regulations, guidelines, and policy statements or statutes.
   1. Regulations can be used to determine the length of time that an opiate may be prescribed, how many units may be delivered, and the procedure by which opiates may be prescribed. Eighteen states currently have regulations that control the distribution of opiates within the respective jurisdictions. (A number of states have laws that mandate triplicate prescriptions for the prescribing of CII medications.) This practice, in and of itself, produces a chilling effect on the prescribing of opiates.
   2. Guidelines and policy statements are less formal and provide parameters for what the state board considers acceptable practice standards when evaluating the use of controlled substances. Guidelines may take the form of the model guidelines published by the Federation of State Medical Boards (1998), or they may be individually crafted to produce the outcome desired by that state. Thirty-two states currently have guidelines and policy statements in place.
   3. Statutes dictate the manner and process that control the practice of pain management within a given jurisdiction and have the legal force and effect of law. Statutes are generally considered to be the most forceful of the three and tend to institutionalize the practice of pain management. Many state statutes follow the Model Intractable Pain Treatment Acts (IPTAs), some progeny of which have been adopted by 22 states. The main goal of these laws is to address physician reluctance to prescribe opiates for the treatment of chronic pain, because of concern about regulatory scrutiny, by providing immunity from discipline by state medical boards when certain diagnostic criteria are met. Although the creation of IPTAs was stimulated by interest in chronic noncancer pain, most IPTAs nevertheless apply to prescribing for intractable pain, including prescribing for patients with cancer or AIDS.

Civil Proceedings

Malpractice, if it has been asserted with a reasonable degree of certainty, may result in a civil tort action. An action to strip a license by a state medical board would be a powerful tool for the plaintiff in this type of litigation. It is important to note, however, that inaction by a state board does not necessarily serve as an affirmative defense should an action in negligence be brought against a caregiver.

A. Civil proceedings for inadequate treatment of pain fall under a charge of negligence. Plaintiffs must assert and prove the four prima facie elements to win an action for professional negligence.
1. The provider owed a duty of care to the patient.
2. That duty was breached in a manner that materially disaffected the patient.
3. The patient's injury was proximately caused by the provider's negligence.
4. Damages accrued to the patient because the provider failed in his or her discharge of the duty to the patient.

B. No state currently recognizes failure to treat pain as a cause of action, but
1. A North Carolina nursing home was assessed a $15 million judgment for allowing a patient to die writhing in pain (*Estate of Henry James v. Hillhaven Corp.,* 1990).
2. More than 50 plaintiff actions have been identified that are alleging a failure to treat pain.
3. Reports in the popular press show trends of increasing jury awards for elder neglect in nursing homes and other venues ("Getting Sued," 1998; "Jury Awards," 1995; "Nursing Home Verdicts," 1998).

C. The JCAHO standards that became effective on January 1, 2001, established a threshold for adequate pain management. With this regulation in place, it is now empirically possible to assess a caregiver's treatment of pain against a recognized accepted and mandated standard of care (Rich, 2000). Thus, it can be stated that a duty is now recognized on the part of the caregiver to effectively manage and reduce a patient's pain wherever medically possible.

References

Drug Enforcement Administration. (1970). *Controlled Substances Act.* Washington, DC: Author.

Estate of Henry James v. Hillhaven Corp. (1990). Sup. Ct. Div. 89CVS64, Hertford County, NC.

Federation of State Medical Boards. (1998). *Model guidelines for the use of controlled substances for the treatment of pain.* Retrieved October 22, 2001 from the World Wide Web: http://www.fsmb.org

Getting sued by seniors. (1998, December). *ABA Journal,* pp. 28–29.

Joranson, D.E., & Gilson, A.M. (2001). Pharmacists' knowledge and attitudes toward opioid pain medication in relation to federal and state policies. *Journal of the American Pharmaceutical Association, 41,* 213–220.

Jury awards rise for improper care of the elderly. (1995, September 5). *Wall Street Journal,* p. B1.

Nursing home verdicts: There's guilt all round. (1998, July 27). *Newsweek,* p. 34.

Rich, B.A. (2000). *A prescription for pain: The emerging standard of care for pain management.* St. Paul, MN: William Mitchell Law Review.

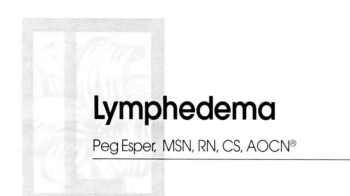

Lymphedema

Peg Esper, MSN, RN, CS, AOCN®

Definition

Lymphedema is an undesired accumulation of lymphatic fluid in tissues as a result of increased production of lymphatic fluid or an obstruction of lymphatic flow.

Pathophysiology/Etiology

A number of conditions may result in the development of chronic lymphedema. Patients who have undergone surgical excision of lymph nodes are at a higher risk of developing lymphedema because of an alteration of lymphatic flow. When tumor blocks lymphatic drainage in the subcutaneous tissues, obstruction can lead to lymphedema. Surgery can result in significant scarring and subsequent obstruction of flow. Immobility in patients who are terminally ill also leads to diminished skeletal muscle contraction and decreased ability to move lymph fluid through lymphatic channels. Excessive lymphedema can adversely affect a patient's quality of life by causing pain and fatigue, decreasing mobility, and having negative effects on body image (Smith & Zobec, 2001).

Manifestations

- Swelling of affected limb
- Heaviness
- Pain
- Burning
- Fatigue
- Erythema
- Cellulitis
- Decreased mobility

Management

A. General measures

1. Assess the degree of lymphedema now and over the last few months.
2. Identify current measures being used to manage the lymphedema.
3. Evaluate affected extremity for evidence of infection, and institute treatment as appropriate ($)—cephalexin (Keflex®) 500 mg po tid–qid x 14 days (Kalinowski, 1999).
4. Attempt to keep extremity elevated as much as possible.

B. Death is not imminent.
   1. Use of compression garments ($–$$)—elastic bandages or compression stockings (Badger, Peacock, & Mortimer, 2000)
   2. Use of compression pumps ($$$)—not always effective, pressure no greater than 60 mm Hg (Smith & Zobec, 2001)
   3. Use of massage therapy—patient/caregivers can be instructed by physical therapist or lymphedema specialist to perform this themselves (Finlay, 1999)
   4. Complex decongestive physiotherapy ($$$)—a series of five techniques that are combined as an intense approach to the management of lymphedema. The techniques consist of
      a) Skin care to prevent infection
      b) Specialized massage
      c) Bandaging with nonelastic bandages
      d) Exercises performed while bandages are in place, followed by application of a compression garment (Kalinowski, 1999; Smith & Zobec).
   5. The use of diuretics generally is not recommended, as they tend to pull fluid out of the vasculature and not out of the tissue spaces, leading to complaints of dizziness, lightheadedness, and hypotension (Smith & Zobec).
   6. Analgesic support for pain symptoms (See Pain.)
   7. Increase protein in diet as tolerated.

C. Death is imminent.
   1. The application of compression garments or use of massage and wraps at this point should be determined on an individual-patient basis.
   2. No long-term benefits are available for the patient, and continuation of measures actually may increase discomfort.
   3. The goal of care should be directed at alleviating any discomfort caused by the lymphedema and assisting the patient with movement as needed.

Patient Outcomes

A. Optimal control of lymphedema

B. Optimal comfort when lymphedema cannot be resolved

Professional Competencies

A. Identify factors that place the patient at risk for the development of lymphedema.

B. Identify measures to decrease lymphedema.

C. Demonstrate appropriate level of aggressive treatment based on individual patient condition.

Measurement Instruments

A. Measuring the affected extremity on a regular basis with measuring tape

B. Quality-of-life measurement

C. Functional assessment (See Fatigue.)

References

Badger, C., Peacock, J., & Mortimer, P. (2000). A randomized, controlled, parallel-group clinical trial comparing multilayer bandaging followed by hosiery versus hosiery alone in the treatment of patients with lymphedema of the limb. *Cancer, 88,* 2832–2837.

Finlay, I. (1999). End-of-life care in patients dying of gynecologic cancer. *Hematology/Oncology Clinics of North America, 13,* 77–108.

Kalinowski, B.H. (1999). Lymphedema. In C. Yarbro, M. Frogge, & M. Goodman (Eds.), *Cancer symptom management* (pp. 457–466). Boston: Jones and Bartlett.

Smith, J.K., & Zobec, A. (2001). Lymphedema. In B. Ferrell & N. Coyle (Eds.), *Textbook of palliative nursing* (pp. 192–203). New York: Oxford University Press.

Nausea and Vomiting

Mellar Davis, MD, FCCP

Definition

Nausea is the unpleasant sensation of the need to vomit and is associated with diaphoresis, lightheadedness, and pallor. Retching follows the spasmodic movement of the diaphragm and abdominal musculature; when combined with pyloric and lower esophageal relaxation followed by retroperistalsis, vomiting occurs (Davis & Walsh, 2000; Twycross & Back, 1998).

Pathophysiology/Etiology

Sixty percent of terminally ill patients have nausea unrelated to antitumor therapy, and 30% vomit (Komurcu, Nelson, & Walsh, 2000). Both are demoralizing, demeaning, and significantly reduce the quality of life. Nausea detrimentally contributes to anorexia and accelerates weight loss, further reducing the patient's performance abilities and accentuating fatigue (Carney & Meier, 2000; Davis & Walsh, 2000). Patients with advanced diseases frequently are on a multitude of potentially emetogenic medications. These include antibiotics, digoxin, nonsteroidal anti-inflammatory agents, anticonvulsants, opiates, and iron. Advanced malignancies are associated with autonomic failure, early satiety, and nausea independent of antitumor therapy (Carney & Meier; Twycross & Back, 1998). Depression and anxiety can induce gastroparesis and nausea. Morning nausea with focal neurologic changes suggests posterior fossa tumors. Crampy abdominal pain, bloating, and large-volume vomitus herald bowel obstruction. Postprandial nausea with vomiting and no nausea between meals suggest a gastric outlet obstruction or severe gastroparesis (Davis & Walsh). Hyperglycemia and hypercalcemia induce gastroparesis, accompanied by polydipsia, nausea, polyuria, and vomiting. Uremia and hyponatremia produce neurologic changes, somnolence with nausea, resembling brain secondaries. Iatrogenic Addison's crisis produces asthenia with nausea and occurs secondary to abrupt discontinuation of progesterone or corticosteroids.

Manifestations

- Stomatitis
- Organomegaly
- Ascites
- High-pitched bowel sounds
- Abdominal distension
- Rectal impaction
- Anorexia
- Hypercalcemia
- Papilledema (central nervous system malignancy)

(Davis & Walsh, 2000; Mannix, 1998; Twycross & Back, 1998)

Management

A. Important questions to ask patients who are experiencing nausea
   1. When did the nausea begin?
   2. What has been tried to relieve nausea, and what makes the nausea worse?
   3. What is the appearance of the vomitus, and what is the volume?
   4. Is there colic or abdominal pain?
   5. Where is the location of pain and its character?
   6. When was the last bowel movement?
   7. Is there abdominal distention or bloating?
   8. Is the patient passing flatus?
   9. Is the nausea associated with meals or medications?
   10. Has there been any recent form of treatment?

B. Death is not imminent.
   1. Treat the underlying cause when possible (Davis & Walsh, 2000; Mannix, 1998; Twycross & Back, 1998).
      a) Hypercalcemia—Bisphosphonates, calcitonin ($$)
      b) Central nervous system disease
          (1) Steroids ($) for increased intracranial pressure
          (2) Radiation therapy ($$$$) for newly diagnosed metastatic disease
      c) Modify medications if contributing to nausea/vomiting
      d) See Ascites.
      e) See Bowel Obstruction.
      f) See Depression.
      g) See Infection (note measures regarding the oral cavity).
      h) See Pain.
   2. If underlying cause is unknown or untreatable (Burger, 2001)
      a) Nonpharmacologic treatment
          (1) Avoid greasy, fatty foods.
          (2) Keep a small amount of food in the stomach at all times.

    (3) Increase salty foods (saltines), fresh foods, broth, and cold foods.
    (4) Avoid strong odors or bothersome smells.
    (5) Practice distraction, guided imagery, or hypnosis.
    (6) Use acupressure.
    (7) Use aromatherapy (peppermint).
    (8) Take ginger tea.
    (9) Rehydrate with IV fluids to help break cyclic nausea and vomiting and related dehydration ($$).
  b) Pharmacologic treatment (Cole, Robinson, Harvey, Trethowan, & Murdoch, 1994; Davis & Walsh; Mannix; Twycross & Back)
    (1) A number of agents can be used alone or in combination to block nausea and vomiting (see Table 1).

Table 1. Antiemetic Agents

Classification	Dose/Routes
Anticholinergics	
Glycopyrrolate (Robinul®) ($)	0.2 mg sq q6h
Hyoscyamine sulfate (Levsin®) ($)	0.125 mg po/sl q8h
Scopolamine (Transderm-Scop®) ($$)	0.2–0.4 mg sq q4h; one patch q3 days
Benzodiazepine	
Lorazepam (Ativan®) ($)	$1–1.5$ mg/m^2 IV q4–6h
	1–2 mg po/sl q3–4h
Butyrophenone	
Haloperidol (Haldol®) ($)	0.5–5.0 mg po/IV q6–8h
Cannabinoid	
Dronabinol (Marinol®) ($$)	2.5–10.0 mg po q4–6h
Corticosteroid	
Dexamethasone (Decadron®) ($)	2–8 mg po/IV q6–8h
Dopamine antagonist	
Metoclopramide (Reglan®) ($)	10 mg po q6–8h
	10 mg IV q3–4h
Phenothiazenes	
Chlorpromazine (Thorazine®) ($)	10–25 mg po q4h
	50–100 mg pr q6–8h
	25–50 mg IM q4–6h
Olanzapine (Zyprexa®) ($$)	2.5–5.0 mg po q12h
Ondansetron (Zofran®) ($$)	8 mg po/IV/sq q8h
Prochlorperazine (Compazine®) ($–$$)	10 mg po/IM/IV q6h
	25 mg pr q6h
Promethazine (Phenergan®) ($–$$)	12.5–25 mg po/IV/IM/pr q4–6h
Trimethobenzamide (Tigan®) ($)	250 mg po q6–8h
	200 mg pr/IM q6h

Note. Based on information from Carney et al., 2000; Mannix, 1998.

        (2) Severe nausea/vomiting: Two to five of the following agents may be compounded as suppositories or troches for the patient with very difficult to control nausea and vomiting (Burger, 2001).

           (a) Lorazepam (Ativan®)
           (b) Diphenhydramine (Benadryl®)
           (c) Haloperidol (Haldol®)
           (d) Metoclopramide (Reglan®)
           (e) Dexamethasone (Decadron®)
           (f) Droperidol (Inapsine®)
           (g) Ondansetron (Zofran®)

C. Death is imminent (Davis & Walsh, 2000).
1. Patients in their last two weeks of life often develop delirium, complete anorexia, and may be bedfast.
2. Extensive investigations using radiographic procedures are inappropriate.
3. The bedside clinician should focus on symptom control.
4. Terminal delirium may appear with nausea, both requiring treatment.
5. Choosing agents that treat two symptoms at one time is wise prescribing.
    a) Chlorpromazine (Thorazine®) treats both terminal delirium and nausea while being very inexpensive compared to benzodiazepines (e.g., lorazepam plus haloperidol).
    b) Haloperidol (Haldol®) has multiple routes of administration (IV, sq, and po), and chlorpromazine is given either IV, po, or per rectum.
    c) Gastric suctioning by nasogastric tube may be necessary in patients with a terminal bowel obstruction; PEG tubes and stenting are not attempted and are inappropriate at this stage of illness.
    d) The use of high-dose IV antiemetics/sedatives may be required to achieve control of symptoms.

Patient Outcomes

A. Relief of nausea and vomiting

B. Tolerates small amounts of food/fluids at a time

Professional Competencies

A. Identify the underlying cause of nausea and vomiting when possible and institute measures to correct it.

B. Identify pharmacologic and nonpharmacologic measures to control nausea and vomiting.

C. Evaluate effectiveness of treatment plan, and modify as appropriate.

References

Burger, T. (2001). Pain and symptom management. In B. Poor & G. Poirrier (Eds.), *End-of-life nursing care* (pp. 139–174). Boston: Jones and Bartlett.

Carney, M., & Meier, D. (2000). Palliative care and end of life issues. *Anesthesiology Clinics of North America, 18,* 183–208.

Cole, R., Robinson, F., Harvey, L., Trethowan, K., & Murdoch, V. (1994). Successful control of intractable nausea and vomiting requiring combined ondansetron and haloperidol in a patient with advanced cancer. *Journal of Pain and Symptom Management, 9,* 48–50.

Davis, M.P., & Walsh, D. (2000). Treatment of nausea and vomiting in advanced cancer. *Supportive Care in Cancer, 8,* 444–452.

Komurcu, S., Nelson, K.A., & Walsh, D. (2000). The gastrointestinal symptoms of advanced cancer. *Supportive Care in Cancer, 9,* 32–39.

Mannix, K. (1998). Palliation in nausea and vomiting. In D. Doyle, G.W.C. Hanks, & N. MacDonald (Eds.), *Oxford textbook of palliative medicine* (2nd ed.) (pp. 489–499). New York: Oxford University Press.

Twycross, R., & Back, I. (1998). Nausea and vomiting in advanced cancer. *European Journal of Palliative Care, 5,* 39–45.

Pain

Marco Pappagallo, MD, E. Duke Dickerson, MSc,
PhD, James Varga, RPh, MBA, Joshua M. Cox, RPh,
Costantino Benedetti, MD, Mellar Davis, MD, FCCP,
and Peg Esper, MSN, RN, CS, AOCN®

Definition

Pain is one of the most common symptoms experienced by patients with advanced cancer. The International Association for the Study of Pain (IASP) defines pain as an unpleasant sensory and emotional experience associated with actual or potential tissue damage or described in terms of such damage (IASP, 1979). Pain may be acute or chronic and also occurs in the unresponsive patient. Patients also may have "breakthrough" pain. *Breakthrough pain* refers to a transient exacerbation of pain outside of what has been experienced by the individual in a "controlled" pain state.

Pathophysiology/Etiology

The fear of being in pain remains one of the most prevalent concerns for patients with advanced illnesses (Twycross, 1999). Educating patients, caregivers, and healthcare providers about pain is critical. Most pain experienced by adult patients with cancer is a direct result of cancer, a small percentage is related to treatment, and less than 10% is linked to cancer-related debility (e.g., constipation, muscle spasm) and concurrent disorders (e.g., osteoarthritis). All patients with advanced illnesses are at risk of developing a variety of pain syndromes that have similar management approaches, regardless of whether the pain is malignant or nonmalignant (Esper, 2000).

Manifestations

Manifestations are determined by the type and site of pain experienced. Three general categories include somatic, visceral, and neuropathic.

Somatic Pain

Nociceptive pains related to ongoing activation of somatic primary afferents also are termed somatic pains. These pains typically are described as aching, squeezing, stabbing, or throbbing. Arthritis and some types of cancer pain (e.g., bone pain) exemplify somatic nociceptive pains. The hallmark of somatic nociceptive pain is an aching quality that is exacerbated by movement or weight bearing (Kanner, 1996).

Visceral Pain

Visceral pain results from stimulation of afferent sensory fibers that follow sympathetic nerves in the thoracic and lumbar paravertebral ganglia and is evoked by obstruction, perforation, and distension of hollow organs (Cervero & Laird, 1999). Visceral pain is diffuse, poorly localized, and accompanied by intense motor and autonomic reflexes. Visceral pain is associated with colic, which is episodic, relatively opiate resistant, and nonpositional.

Neuropathic Pain

Neuropathic cancer pain can be caused by direct tumor infiltration of neural structures or secondary effects produced by treatment of the underlying neoplasm. Neuropathic pain results from dysfunction of or injury to the peripheral nervous system or the central nervous system (Woolf & Mannion, 1999). Neuropathic cancer pain is almost always associated with sensory changes. Patients with neuropathic pain usually present with a spontaneous ongoing or intermittent pain typically characterized by a burning or shooting electric-shock quality. Neuropathic pain can present one of the greatest challenges in providing optimal pain control. Appendix A has been devoted to an in-depth advanced review of the management of neuropathic pain.

Pain Assessment and Evaluation

Assessment of pain includes learning about location, intensity, radiation, palliative and exacerbating factors, as well as quality of pain. The patients' description of their pain may need to be prompted by a series of questions. The mnemonic PQRST can be helpful in interviewing patients.

Palliative factors—What makes your pain better?

Provocative factors—What makes your pain worse?

Quality—What exactly is it like?

Radiation—Does it spread anywhere?

Severity—How severe is it?

Temporal factors—How much does the pain affect your life?

A visual analog scale often is used to assist in quantifying the severity of pain a patient is experiencing.

Management

Management of pain involves very specific goals. These include finding the agent(s) that will control pain at an established level acceptable to the patient. The regimen of choice is the one with the fewest side effects that allows for optimal functional status and is feasible for the patient to take based on factors related to absorption, availability, tolerability, and cost. This section has not been divided to reflect intervention based on the patient's proximity to death, to avoid unnecessary repetition. However, those interventions with a * symbol generally are not considered to be appropriate when death is imminent (see Table 1).

A. Barriers to pain management (Benedetti, Dickerson, & Nicholls, 2001; Esper, 2000; Oneschuk, Hanson, & Bruera, 2000)
   1. Inexperience and lack of education on the part of healthcare providers
   2. Fear of addiction (patients, family members, and healthcare providers)
   3. Concern of patients that they need to delay using analgesics so that their pain will not be uncontrollable when they are closer to death

B. Eliminate the cause of pain when possible (see Table 1).

Table 1. Pain Interventions by Source of Pain

Source of Pain	Intervention
Metastatic lesions in bone	• Radiation therapy ($$$$)* • Radioisotope injection ($$$$)* • Bisphosphonates ($$)* • Immobilization of affected area
Inflammation from infected wounds or tissues	Antibiotic therapy ($–$$) (See Infection.)
Enlarging masses putting pressure on adjacent structures	• Radiation therapy ($$$$)* • Chemotherapy ($$–$$$$)* • Tumor embolization ($$$)* • Nerve block ($$$)* (e.g., celiac block in the individual with pancreatic cancer)

C. Therapeutic intervention: A number of pharmacologic and nonpharmacologic measures can be considered when the cause of pain cannot be determined or eliminated.
   1. Pharmacologic interventions
      a) Mild pain—nonopiate analgesics
         (1) Nonsteroidal anti-inflammatory drugs (NSAIDs) (Motrin®, Advil®) ($–$$)—block biosynthesis of prostaglandin with anti-inflammatory effects
         (2) Acetaminophen (Tylenol®) ($)—central nervous system inhibition of prostaglandin but without anti-inflammatory properties
            (a) Around-the-clock dosing is preferred.
            (b) Administer NSAIDs with food to prevent gastrointestinal irritation.
      b) Moderate pain

(1) Opiate analgesic with or without nonopiate analgesic (Benedetti & Dickerson, 1999)

(2) Comparative analgesic properties of common opiates used in pain management (see Table 2)

Table 2. Comparative Analgesic Table

Agent	Equivalent Dosing to Oral Morphine 15 mg q4h	Maximum Daily Dose
Codeine ($)	100 mg q4h	None
Fentanyl TTS ($$$$)	25 mcg/h	None
Hydromorphone NR ($$)	4 mg q4h	None
Methadone ($)	5 mg q6–8h or 10 mg q8h	None
Morphine SR ($$$)	30 mg q8h or 45 mg q12h	None
Oxycodone NR ($$)	15 mg q4h	None
Oxycodone SR ($$$$$)	30 mg q8h or 45 mg q12h	None
Tramadol ($$$$)	100 mg q6h	400 mg

NR = normal release; SR = sustained release; TTS = transdermal
Note. For opiate-tolerant patients, there is no recognized ceiling dose. As the dose is raised, analgesic effects increase in a log-linear function until either analgesia is achieved or side effects occur. In practice, the efficacy of any particular opiate in a specific patient will be determined by the degree of analgesia produced following dose escalation through a range that is limited by the development of side effects (Cherny, 1996).

(3) Sustained-release agents should be initiated when the patient's normal release dosing requirements have been titrated rapidly enough to control the patient's pain.

(4) Breakthrough pain medication should be readily available for patients on long-acting/sustained-release agents (dosing should be 10%–20% of the long-acting dose).

(5) If breakthrough pain exceeds three or four episodes per day or consistently awakens the patient during the night, consider an increase in the dosage of the long-acting agent.

c) Severe pain often requires increased doses of opiates as well as the possibility of the addition of invasive routes of administration.

(1) Subcutaneous or intravenous administration ($$–$$$$)

(a) A variety of delivery methods (injection, subcutaneous buttons, pumps, peripherally inserted central catheter [PICC] lines) are available and can be very effective in providing increased concentrations of opiate analgesics with a steady rate of delivery.

(b) Bolus dosing also is possible with these routes of administration.

(c) Side effects are the same as seen in oral administration but may be increased because of an increased dosage of agents.

(2) Epidural/intrathecal administration ($$$$)

(a) Less medication is required, which often means decreased side effects; however, more sophisticated monitoring is required.

(b) If implantable pumps are used, they must be removed at the time of death for patients wishing to be cremated.

d) Adjuvant agents—Many agents can be used in conjunction with nonopiate and opiate analgesics to augment pain relief. Their primary indication is not generally for analgesia, but when combined with opiates, they often can optimize pain relief (see Table 3).

(1) Anticonvulsant drugs (ACDs) (e.g., carbamazapine [Tegretol®], gabapentin [Neurontin®], lamotrigine [Lamictal®]) ($$)—ACDs are common analgesic adjuvants to treat neuropathic pain. These agents are recommended as first-line adjuvants of neuropathic pain incompletely responding to opiate treatment.

(2) Antidepressants (e.g., tricyclics, selective serotonin reuptake inhibitors) ($–$$)—Antidepressants have been found to be useful in helping manage neuropathic pain even when patients are not clinically depressed. The tricyclic antidepressants have been used longer than other classifications of these agents, but newer agents should not be overlooked as a possible addition to the pain management armamentarium.

Table 3. Analgesic Adjuvants

Agent	Starting Dose
Anticonvulsants	
Carbamazepine (Tegretol®)	100–200 mg po q12h
Gabapentin (Neurontin®)	300 mg po q8h
Lamotrigine (Lamictal®)	25 mg po q12h
Tricyclic antidepressants	
Amitriptyline (Elavil®)	25 mg po qhs
Desipramine (Norpramin®)	25–75 mg po qhs
Nortriptyline (Pamelor®)	25 mg po qhs
Corticosteroids	
Dexamethasone (Decadron®)	4–16 mg po qam
Prednisone (Deltasone®)	5–10 mg po qam
Cannabinoid	
Dronabinol (Marinol®)	2.5–5.0 mg po qhs or q8h
Bisphosphonate	
Pamidronate (Aredia®)	60–90 mg IV over 3–4h q3–4 wk
Zolendronate (Zometa®)	4 mg IV over 15 minutes
Miscellaneous	
Mexiletine (Mexitil®)	150 mg po q8h

(3) Corticosteroids ($) (e.g., dexamethasone [Decadron®], prednisone [Deltasone®])—Alternatives to NSAIDs, particularly in patients who have coagulopathies or gastritis that precludes the use of NSAIDs. Corticosteroids uniquely reduce headaches associated with cerebral metastasis and symptoms related to bowel obstruction. Methylprednisolone (Medrol®) can be used with benefit in painful plexopathies caused by cancer infiltration of nerve trunks.

(4) Cannabinoids ($$)—Combinations of low doses of cannabinoids and low doses of opiate mu-agonists (e.g., morphine, hydromorphone [Dilaudid®], methadone [Dolophine®], and fentanyl [Duragesic®]) ($–$$$) produce antinociception.

(5) Bisphosphonates (e.g., pamidronate [Aredia®]) ($$$)—Can reduce bone pain and prevent bone fracture and morbidity in patients with multiple myeloma and breast cancer as well as other metastatic bone disease.

(6) Mexiletine (Mexitil®) ($)—An antiarrhythmic that stabilizes neuronal membranes, reducing neuropathic pain. Mexiletine is a sodium channel blocker whose analgesic mechanism is similar to that of some ACDs. Mexiletine is contraindicated in the patient with cardiac conduction defects or blocks. Gastrointestinal side effects (e.g., diarrhea, nausea) can be significant.

2. Nonpharmacologic interventions

   a) See Complementary Therapies.

   b) Neurosurgical procedures such as neuroablation, nerve blocks, and neurostimulating procedures (transcutaneous nerve stimulation) are beneficial for some patients; these generally require formal consultation to determine potential benefit.

3. Side effects of therapy

   a) Constipation—By far one of the most problematic side effects seen in pain management. Patients should be placed on a bowel regimen at the same time that analgesics are instituted. (See Constipation.)

   b) Nausea—Some analgesics may produce nausea as a side effect. It may be necessary to change to a different analgesic if nausea cannot be controlled adequately. (See Nausea and Vomiting.)

   c) Sedation—Incremental titration of opiate dosing will help to decrease problems with oversedation. It is not uncommon for patients who have experienced significant pain to appear sedated initially after pain is under adequate control, but this should be a temporary phenomenon. The need to use "reversal" agents is rare, and their use should be considered very carefully to prevent significant flares in pain.

Patient Outcomes

A. An acceptable level of pain control is achieved.

B. Optimal management of side effects is achieved.

C. Pain control is achieved without excessive sedation or delirium.

D. Improved quality of life and functional status are attained.

Professional Competencies

A. Accurately assess patient's pain status.

B. Recognize the appropriate use of interventions to control pain as determined by type, severity, comorbidities, and patient preferences.

C. Titrate pain medications to achieve optimal control of pain with the fewest side effects.

D. Ongoing assessment of patient comfort level occurs with adjustment of the plan for optimal control of patient pain and side effects.

E. Both pharmacologic and nonpharmacologic interventions are used as appropriate.

F. Adjuvant medications are used as appropriate to optimize pain management.

Measurement Instruments

A. Numeric rating scales

B. Visual analog scales

C. Categorical scales

D. Faces scale
(National Comprehensive Cancer Network, 2000)

References

Benedetti, C., & Dickerson, E. (1999). Criteria for opioid selection. *Journal of Pain and Symptom Management, 19,* 410–411.

Benedetti, C., Dickerson, E., & Nicholls, L. (2001). Medical education: A barrier in pain therapy and palliative care. *Journal of Pain and Symptom Management, 21,* 360–362.

Cervero, F., & Laird, J. (1999). Visceral pain. *Lancet, 353,* 2145–2148.

Cherny, N. (1996). Opioid analgesics: Comparative features and prescribing guidelines. *Drugs, 51,* 713–737.

Esper, P. (2000). Pain management in patients with advanced malignancies. *Home Health Consultant, 7,* 11–18.

International Association for the Study of Pain. (1979). Subcommittee on Taxonomy of Pain Terms. A list with definitions and notes on usage. *Pain, 6,* 249.

Kanner, R. (1996). Low back pain. In R.K. Portenoy, & R.M. Kanner (Eds.), *Pain management: Theory and practice* (p.135). Philadelphia: F.A. Davis Company.

National Comprehensive Cancer Network. (2000). *NCCN practice guidelines for cancer pain.* Rockledge, PA: Author.

Oneschuk, D., Hanson, J., & Bruera, E. (2000). An International Survey of Undergraduate Medical Education in Palliative Medicine. *Journal of Pain and Symptom Management, 20,* 174–179.

Twycross, R. (1999). *Introducing palliative care* (3rd ed.). Abingdon, England: Radcliffe Medical Press.

Woolf, C., & Mannion, R. (1999). Neuropathic pain: Aetiology, symptoms, mechanisms, and management. *Lancet, 353,* 1959–1964.

Palliative Care

Helen K. McHale, MSN, RN, CHPN

Definition

Palliative care is the active total care provided to patients living with advanced incurable illness and their families. The focus of care shifts to quality of life and the alleviation of distressing symptoms versus aggressive biomedical interventions. The goal of palliative care is neither to hasten nor postpone death. It provides relief from pain and other distressing symptoms and integrates the psychologic and spiritual aspects of care. Furthermore, it offers a support system to help relatives and friends cope during the patient's illness and bereavement (National Coalition on Health Care, 2001).

Specific Issues Related to Palliative Care

Aging of the U.S. Population

More attention is being given to managing and living with advanced illness and recognizing the limits and inappropriate use of technologic resources. Societal demands for assisted suicide and public apprehensions about suffering at the end of life are frequently raised issues.

Unnecessary Life-Prolonging Technology

This has contributed to a renewed interest in humane end-of-life care. Increased awareness of the success of hospice as an alternative model of care has served as a catalyst for integrating palliative care into traditional models of healthcare delivery.

Palliative Care Is a Clinical Specialty

Palliative care acknowledges that dying is a normal part of living. Although a new entity of Western practice, palliative care is a well-defined medical specialty that combines an interdisciplinary approach to promote competent and compassionate care. It is the vision that palliative care becomes the standard of care for Americans living with life-limiting illness.

Focus of Palliative Care

Palliative care is patient- and family-centered. It
- Provides physical comfort and emotional support
- Promotes shared medical/nursing decision making
- Treats each person as an individual by understanding his or her needs and expectations
- Attends to the needs of those who care for and love the dying person (National Coalition on Health Care, 2001).

Levels of Palliative Care

Palliative care consists of three levels, each identifying prescribed treatments and goals. From the following levels, note that levels I and II treat the disease, whereas level III focuses more readily on medical futility, and the shift in treatment promotes the philosophy of comfort up to and until the time of death.

Level I:
- The goal is to prolong survival by arresting the disease process.
- Patients are willing and physically able to tolerate side effects associated with treatment (e.g., chemotherapy, radiation, surgery).
- The psychoemotional goal for the patient is to fight the disease and to live as long as possible.

Level II:
- The goal is to treat the tumor or the disease to improve symptoms.
- Patients are willing and physically able to tolerate minimal side effects associated with treatment.
- The psychoemotional goal for the patient is the achievement of hope.

Level III:
- The goal is to achieve a satisfactory level of comfort for the patient.
- Patients become unwilling and are unable to tolerate the side effects associated with aggressive interventions.
- The psychoemotional goal is to surrender and accept the disease process (Heidrich, 1999).

Strategies to Promote Quality Palliative Care

A. Educate healthcare providers to overcome barriers to competent palliative care.
   1. End-of-life discussions are required because of the negative connotations associated with death.
   2. Patients and their families are to be informed about advance directives.
   3. Referring patients to hospice or palliative care does not mean giving up control over patients.
   4. Reimbursement for the time healthcare professionals spend consulting with terminally ill patients and families is available.

5. Patients and families may not be accepting the diagnosis of an incurable illness (Tobin & Larson, 2001).

B. Palliative care should be offered to patients when illness becomes incurable.
   1. It may be difficult to decide when patients are appropriate for palliative care.
   2. If the question "Is this patient ill enough that you would not be surprised if he or she died in the next year?" is answered affirmatively, the patient is eligible for palliative services (National Coalition on Health Care & Institute for Healthcare Improvement, 2000).

C. Assessing the terminal phase
   1. Experienced providers describe the importance of recognizing patient deterioration.
   2. Changes in the patient's condition may signal a shift from a chronic to a terminal phase of illness.
   3. Ongoing assessment for signs of deterioration should initiate end-of-life discussions.
   4. The following conditions often distinguish the terminal phase of an illness (Norton & Talerico, 2000).
      a) Worsening symptoms, especially shortness of breath, fatigue, confusion, and pain
      b) Loss of appetite
      c) Weight loss
      d) Increased frequency or severity of exacerbations
      e) Decreased activity tolerance
      f) Increased use of assistive devices
      g) Talk of death
      h) Finishing business
      i) Talking to dead relatives
      j) Withdrawal

Patient Outcomes

A. Articulates information regarding diagnosis and prognosis

B. Receives care that reflects continuity, coordination, and comprehension of the disease trajectory

C. Remains informed of expected symptoms and how to manage them effectively

D. Receives customized care based upon personal preferences and available resources (National Coalition on Health Care & Institute for Healthcare Improvement, 2000)

Professional Competencies

Delayed or inadequate planning may have profound negative consequences for patients, families, or their providers. Strategies to facilitate end-of-life decision making include (Norton & Talerico, 2000)

A. Appropriate communication regarding patient condition
1. Be willing to both initiate and engage in discussions about end-of-life issues.
2. Use words such as *death* and *dying* in discussions with patients and their families.
3. Be specific when discussing what there is hope for (e.g., "a good death," pain control).
4. Clarify goals and burdens of treatment and prognosis.
5. Collaborate with other providers to give consistent information.

B. Accurate assessment of patient/family needs regarding care
1. Identify changes in the patient's condition that may signal a shift to a terminal phase.
2. Provide timely and factual information to patients and family members regarding the patient's condition.
3. Assist patient/family in determining whether goals are achievable or realistic.

Measurement Instruments

A. The Edmonton Symptoms Assessment System and the Edmonton Comfort Assessment Form, as well as links to other useful tools, are available from the Edmonton Palliative Care Program: www.palliative.org.

B. The Hospice Quality of Life Index and a search engine to access more than 803 quality-of-life instruments applicable across the lifespan are available at the multilingual site of Marcello Tamburino, PhD, at www.qlmed.org/url.htm.

C. The Missoula-Vitas Quality of Life Index, a measurement tool for assessing quality of life during the final stages of terminal illness, is available at www .dyingwell.com/mvqoli.htm.

D. The Palliative Care Outcome Scale (POS), by Professor Irene Higginson, was developed to assess outcomes of palliative care, including the quality of life and care of patients and families. The POS is available in two formats, a staff questionnaire and a patient questionnaire, each containing 12 questions. They can be located at www2.edc.org/lastacts/archives/archivesJan00/POS.asp.

E. Toolkit of Instruments to Measure Care at the End of Life, by Joan Teno, MD, are instruments created to measure the quality of care and life for dying patients and their families; among those is the After-Death Bereavement Family Interview in versions for hospices, nursing, and medicine: www.gwu.edu/~cicd/toolkit/toolkit.htm.

References

Heidrich, D. (1999). *Hospice and palliative nursing certification review course.* West Chester, OH: Bell Tower Publishing.

National Coalition on Health Care. (2001). *New validated instruments: Patient-focused, family-centered care.* Retrieved June 25, 2001 from the World Wide Web: http://www.chcr.brown.edu/pcoc/newvalidatedinstrum.htm

National Coalition on Health Care & Institute for Healthcare Improvement. (2000). *Accelerating change today (ACT) for America's health.* Washington, DC: Author.

Norton, S.A., & Talerico, K.A. (2000). Facilitating end-of-life decision-making: Strategies for communicating and assessing. *Journal of Gerontological Nursing, 26,* 6.

Tobin, D., & Larson, D. (2001, January 16). EOL issues continue to get major press coverage. *Hospice News Network, 5,* p. 3.

Pruritus

Peg Esper, MSN, RN, CS, AOCN®

Definition

Pruritus is a sensation in the skin that may be perceived as a mild irritation or tickling to a very unpleasant itching feeling causing severe distress.

Pathophysiology/Etiology

Pruritus can be caused by a localized irritant or seen as the manifestation of a systemic process. Causes of pruritus seen in individuals at the end of life can include dry skin; drug reactions; paraneoplastic syndromes; obstruction of the biliary tree; hypersensitivity reactions; or as a result of treatment with chemotherapy, radiation, or biotherapy agents. The histamine present in mast cells that lie beneath the epidermis is believed to be responsible, in part, for the activation of cutaneous nerves when scratching the skin after an itch occurs. The exact pathophysiology of pruritus is unclear but may be related to a number of chemical reactions, which may include serotonin, prostaglandins, enkephalins, peptides, and substance P (Pittelkow & Loprinzi, 1998; Seiz & Yarbro, 1999).

Manifestations

- Burning
- Itching
- Insomnia
- Pain
- Sense of something crawling on the skin
- Anxiety

Management

A. General measures

1. Attempt to identify a possible source of pruritus. In the case of hypersensitivity reactions, remove the source of the reaction (e.g., change detergents, medications).
2. Examine the skin for evidence of breakdown from scratching and associated signs and symptoms of infection. Determine if a rash exists.
3. For pruritus related to dry skin, use agents to increase moisture, such as baby oil, Eucerin® cream or aloe ($). Avoid any that contain perfumes or alcohol (Kemp, 1999).
4. A cooler environment helps decrease pruritus. Cool, moist compresses over the affected sites may be beneficial.

B. Pharmacologic agents—Agents that have demonstrated an antipruritic effect (Kemp; Pittelkow & Loprinzi, 1998; Seiz & Yarbro, 1999)
1. Steroid preparations (topical or systemic) ($)
2. Antihistamines ($)—diphenhydramine (Benadryl®) 25–50 mg po tid–qid
3. Miscellaneous agents ($)—hydroxyzine hydrochloride (Atarax®) 25 mg po tid–qid; cimetidine (Tagamet®) may be used adjunctively with antihistamines (Regnard & Tempest, 1998).
4. Bile acid sequestrants ($)—cholestyramine (Questran®) 4 g po qid
5. Tricyclic antidepressants ($)

C. Invasive measures—Biliary stent insertion ($$$) may be appropriate for patients with pruritus caused by biliary tree obstruction (Waller & Caroline, 2000).

Patient Outcomes

A. Pruritus is resolved or at a level acceptable to the patient.

B. Patient experiences minimal side effects from medications.

C. Skin is intact and free from infection.

Professional Competencies

A. Recognize pruritus as a symptom that negatively impacts the affects of life in patients with advanced illnesses.

B. Identify possible etiologies of pruritus in the individual patient.

C. Identify approaches to manage pruritus based on identified causes.

D. Evaluate response to treatment and modify the treatment plan as appropriate.

References

Kemp, C. (1999). *Terminal illness* (2nd ed.). Philadelphia: J.B. Lippincott.

Pittelkow, M., & Loprinzi, C. (1998). Pruritus and sweating. In D. Doyle, G.W.C. Hanks, & N. MacDonald (Eds.), *Oxford textbook of palliative medicine* (2nd ed.) (pp. 148–158). New York: Oxford University Press.

Regnard, C., & Tempest, S. (1998). *A guide to symptom relief in advanced disease.* Hale, England: Hochland & Hochland.

Seiz, A., & Yarbro, C. (1999). Pruritus. In C. Yarbro, M. Frogge, & M. Goodman (Eds.), *Cancer symptom management* (pp. 148–158). Boston: Jones and Bartlett.

Waller, A., & Caroline, N. (2000). *Handbook of palliative care in cancer* (2nd ed.). Boston: Butterworth-Heinemann.

Psychologic Support

Karen J. Stanley, RN, MSN, AOCN®, FAAN

Definition

Very few people are prepared to face the loss of either a loved one or their own mortality. The process of living and dying requires emotional and existential support simultaneously. The dying process often is a climactic experience and, despite patient and family coping skills, will require the gentle transition from skilled interdisciplinary clinicians.

Specific Issues Related to Palliative Care
Interindividual and Varied Coping Skills

The interdisciplinary palliative care team brings specialized skills to help dying patients and their families face what may be the most challenging event of their lives. Identification of underlying emotional issues that interfere with the patient's comfort requires ongoing attention (e.g., identification of a history of substance use to cope is an important element to uncover and will help direct the plan of care).

Difficult Articulation of Emotional or Existential Concerns

The constant demands on the patient's psychologic well-being to continually meet the challenges of advanced illness often are overwhelming to the patient and his or her family. The patient may not be able to identify the emergent emotional changes or issues that underlie physical discomforts. Cultural, religious, intellectual, and familial influences, along with personal values, all have an impact on the patient's interpretation of illness and death (Bush, 1998).

Strategies to Maintain Psychologic Support

A. Consistent and ongoing psychologic assessment

1. Frequent assessment of both indirect and direct indices of psychologic well-being is essential when supporting the patient's quality of life.
2. Subjective assessment and frequent open, nonjudgmental conversations with the patient, his or her family, and friends can help provide important data regarding psychologic issues.
3. It is paramount to discern who the patient's support system is—both personal and professional.

B. Do not assume emotional access to the patient and his or her family.
   1. It is not unusual for patients to conceal from a stranger the full extent of their pain, feelings of self-blame, anger, loss, fears about prognosis, and other difficult experiences (Larson & Tobin, 2000).
   2. Allow the patient to direct the course of emotional evaluation.
   3. Gentle offering of "self" will encourage the patient to discuss important issues. This may take several meetings.
   4. Following through with the presence of self, purposeful listening and empathy will help to promote a trusting relationship (Stanley, 2000). Patients often may test clinicians to determine if they are trustworthy, sincere, and genuine.
   5. Never assume that the full interdisciplinary team will be accepted or necessary.

C. Remain open-minded and nonjudgmental. Patients frequently have deeper issues that require professional introspection; after these issues are identified, they require further discussion. This is a very important time for patient-focused issues and should not be confused with the clinician's values, time restraints, or lack of sincere compassion. Routine experiences for the clinician should never discourage the once-in-a-lifetime experience for the patient and his or her family.

D. Provide patient and family-focused care.
   1. Allow time to hear the patient's story.
      a) Provide an opportunity for life review that can be both comforting and healing for all involved.
      b) Life reviews often elicit underlying feelings, such as guilt, regret, denial, and anger.
   2. Encourage patients to maximize their own personal strengths.

E. Assist the patient and family to establish realistic goals.
   1. Maintaining hope in the face of terminal illness is difficult, but attaining realistic goals (e.g., visiting with an old friend for one hour to say goodbye) is not only comforting but helps provide important closure.
   2. Be careful not to promise what cannot be realistically achieved.

F. Acknowledge current and impending losses.

1. The loss of self is a source of great suffering. Patients may look in a mirror and see someone they do not recognize.
2. Loss is a subjective experience; therefore, personal assumptions should be avoided (Corless, 2000).

G. Explore the meaning of illness with the patient and family; this allows incorrect beliefs to surface and provides an opportunity to make appropriate referrals when necessary.

H. Reinforce nonabandonment.
1. One of the greatest fears of the dying person is that he or she will be abandoned because of physiologic disability and functional limitations.
2. Consistently review the plan of care with the patient and his or her family and empower the accomplishment of realistic goals. Remain consistent and involved.

Patient Outcomes

A. Experiences the opportunity to discuss pressing emotional and existential issues with whomever the patient chooses

B. Directs his or her own care

C. Accomplishes realistic goals

Professional Competencies

A. Respond to patients in a nonthreatening, unhurried, and nonjudgmental manner.

B. Recognize when a "good fit" does not exist between therapeutic self and the patient, and withdraw from his or her care.

C. Acknowledge one's own prejudices and personal values that may interfere with specific patients and their families.

D. Step back from the goals established by the healthcare system when the patient does not value them. Help to redirect the plan of care to meet the patient's realistic expectations and knowledge of his or her care.

E. Allow the patient and his or her family to become the central focus of intervention, not just passive recipients of routine care.

References

Bush, N.J. (1998). Coping and adaptation. In R.M. Carroll-Johnson, L.M. Gorman, & N.J. Bush (Eds.), *Psychosocial nursing care along the cancer continuum* (pp. 35–52). Pittsburgh: Oncology Nursing Press.

Corless, I.B. (2000). Bereavement. In B.R. Ferrell & N. Coyle (Eds.), *Textbook of palliative nursing* (pp. 352–362). New York: Oxford University Press.

Larson, D.G., & Tobin, D.R. (2000). End-of-life conversations: Evolving practice and theory. *JAMA, 284,* 1573–1578.

Stanley, K.J. (2000). Silence is not golden: Conversations with the dying. *Clinical Journal of Oncology Nursing, 4,* 34–40.

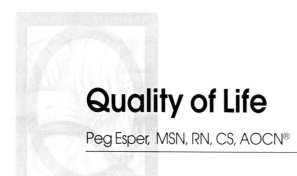

Quality of Life

Peg Esper, MSN, RN, CS, AOCN®

Definition

Quality of life (QOL) is a concept that defines an individual's sense of well-being. QOL is multidimensional and generally believed to include the physical, social, psychologic, and spiritual domains of health and development. These domains are interrelated determinants of the individual's QOL. The ultimate goal of palliative care is to provide an individual with optimal QOL and the subsequent end point of a quality death (Esper & Redman, 1999; King & Hinds, 1998).

Specific Issues Related to Palliative Care

Many issues affect QOL in advanced illness.

Choice to Discontinue Aggressive Treatment

The decision that palliation is the primary goal of care is not to be confused with a "give up" mentality. The hospitalized patient may fear that this decision leads to a room at the end of the hallway where call lights often go unnoticed and staff rounds occur with much less frequency. Even when attention to the physical domain of care may be adequate, the additional needs that relate to QOL may not be addressed. The decision to stop aggressive treatment must not be equated with a decrease in attention to the promotion of optimal QOL (Gorman, 1998).

Symptom Control Versus Maintaining Cognitive Function

A number of the pharmacologic agents used in palliative care for symptom control also may lead to the undesired effects of sedation, somnolence, and altered cognition. Patients may downplay their symptoms because of a fear of becoming oversedated by medications. This negatively impacts their QOL.

Absence of a Multidimensional Approach

Care is sometimes focused on one specific domain of QOL (e.g., physical needs), particularly when the caregiver lacks experience in dealing with the other domains that determine QOL. These domains, however, are interrelated. The physical experience of pain may directly affect the psychologic domain, leading to depression. Unmet psychologic needs may directly affect the individual's ability to experience quality social interactions or impact QOL within the spiritual domain (King & Hinds, 1998).

Limitations Related to Disease Progression

An obvious assault on the individual's QOL is seen as limitations increase with disease progression. A continuum exists within the palliative care period itself, where the goals of care must be consistently reevaluated as the individual is put in the position of taking a more passive role in his or her care (Weinstein, 2001).

Strategies to Promote Optimal Quality of Life

Educate Caregivers on the Needs of Dying Patients

This includes healthcare providers as well as family members. The "avoidance" of terminally ill patients often results from a fear of how to interact with those patients (e.g., what to say, use of touch, what to do if symptoms arise). Increased knowledge of the issues surrounding death and dying can enhance the comfort level of caregivers and ultimately increase patient QOL (Gorman, 1998).

Provide Patients With as Much Control as Possible

Patients must be able to determine what they are willing to endure as far as symptoms are concerned and when relief is more important than cognitive function. Patients and families should be instructed that medications generally can be adjusted to provide optimal relief of signs and symptoms, with minimal effects on the patients' ability to stay in control of their care (Gorman, 1998; Singer, Martin, & Kelner, 1999).

Use a Multidisciplinary Approach to Providing Palliative Care

The healthcare provider's role is to *recognize* the various factors that potentially affect a patient's QOL, not necessarily be the expert in addressing all domains of QOL. QOL is best facilitated when a number of individuals with expertise in varying domains of QOL are available to provide support. A team approach makes the statement that all aspects of QOL are equally important and need to be addressed.

Continuous Reassessment of the Individual's Definition of Quality of Life

The patient's definition of QOL may change frequently during the course of illness. Quality may start out as the ability to go out to a restaurant to enjoy a meal. In the later stages of disease, quality could mean being positioned where he or she can look out a window and view the birds feasting at a bird feeder.

Patient Outcomes

A. Optimal QOL is facilitated through the various stages of the dying process.

B. Autonomy and control are maintained to the extent that is possible.

Professional Competencies

A. Recognize the various domains of QOL.

B. Incorporate a multidisciplinary approach in establishing goals of care for patients.

C. Continually assess the patient's definition of QOL and those interventions to optimize this for the individual.

D. Evaluate the success of measures to improve QOL and modify the plan as appropriate.

Measurement Instruments

Individuals at Brown University have conducted a thorough review of the literature related to instruments developed to measure QOL in palliative care. Their work is available on the World Wide Web at www.chcr.brown.edu/pcoc/quality.htm.

References

Esper, P., & Redman, B. (1999). Supportive care, pain management and quality of life in advanced prostate cancer. *Urologic Clinics of North America, 26*, 375–390.

Gorman, C. (1998). The psychosocial impact of cancer on the individual, family and society. In R.M. Carroll-Johnson, L. Gorman, & N.J. Bush (Eds.), *Psychosocial nursing care along the cancer continuum* (pp. 3–25). Pittsburgh: Oncology Nursing Press.

King, C., & Hinds, P. (1998). *Quality of life: From nursing and patient perspectives.* Boston: Jones and Bartlett.

Singer, P.A., Martin, D.K., & Kelner, M. (1999). Quality end-of-life care. *JAMA, 281*, 163–168.

Weinstein, S. (2001). Integrating palliative care in oncology. *Cancer Control, 8*(1), 32–35.

Seizures

Kimberly A. Zielke, MD

Definition

A recurrent paroxysmal disorder of cerebral function characterized by sudden, brief attacks of altered consciousness, motor activity, or sensory phenomena. The term *status epilepticus* is used when a seizure lasts for more than 30 minutes or recurs at brief intervals, during which the patient does not recover full consciousness (Von Guten, 1999).

Pathophysiology/Etiology

In the terminally ill patient, seizures may be a manifestation of primary brain cancer, cancer that has metastasized to the brain, AIDS, preexisting seizure disorders, metabolic disturbance, or alcohol/drug withdrawal. Witnessing a seizure can be a very frightening experience for both healthcare professionals and family members. Anticipation of seizure potential early in the disease course, with appropriate planning, is necessary for good management (Caracini, 1998).

Manifestations

- Alteration in consciousness
- Dramatic change in consciousness coupled with a fall, tonic-clonic convulsions of all extremities, urinary and fecal incontinence, and amnesia
- Some attacks are preceded by an aura; others provide no warning.
- Muscular contractions of a localized area or only one side of the body
- Myoclonus jerking
- Loss of muscle tone

Management

A. Death is not imminent.

1. Seizures caused by a primary tumor, tumor metastatic to the central nervous system, or to a preexisting condition should be treated with anticonvulsants, such as
   a) Phenobarbital, phenytoin (Dilantin®), or carbamazepine (Tegretol®) ($)
   b) Valproic acid (Depakene®) or gabapentin (Neurontin®) ($$)
   (Dosage should be titrated based on individual needs.)
2. For seizures secondary to a metabolic disturbance (such as hyponatremia, hypercalcemia, or hypoglycemia), consider treating the underlying disturbance; medications contributing to these conditions, such as diuretics or hypoglycemics, need to be decreased in dose or discontinued.
3. All patients at risk for seizures should have medication on hand that would be given in the event that a seizure occurs.
   a) Lorazepam (Ativan®) ($) 1–2 mg sl/sq
   b) Rectal diazepam (Valium®) ($$) 5 mg pr
   c) Lorazepam or midazolam (Versed®) ($$$) sq infusion 30–60 mg/24 hours (Caracini, 1998)

B. Death is imminent: Regardless of the cause, the seizure should be treated with a benzodiazepine such as lorazepam (1–2 mg sl or sc) or a barbiturate (Von Guten, 1999).

Patient Outcomes

A. Prevention of seizures, when possible

B. Quick cessation of seizure

C. Correction of reversible causes of seizures

Professional Competencies

A. Identify patients at high risk for seizures.

B. Identify etiology of seizures and correct, if possible.

C. Facilitate treatment of seizures if they occur.

D. Provide reassurance/support to patient and family members.

E. Identify need for terminal sedation when seizures cannot be readily controlled.

References

Caracini, A. (1998). Neurological problems. In D. Doyle, G.W.C. Hanks, & N. MacDonald (Eds.), *Oxford textbook of palliative medicine* (2nd ed.) (pp. 737–738). New York: Oxford University Press.

Von Guten, C. (1999). Evaluation and management of neuropsychiatric symptoms. In R. Schonwetter (Ed.), *Hospice and palliative medicine* (pp. 103–104). Dubuque, IA: Kendall/ Hunt Publishing.

Sexuality

Beth Cohen, RNC, ARNP, MSN

Definition

Sexuality is the quality of being sexual or the expression of sexual receptivity or interest.

Specific Issues Related to Palliative Care

Sexual response has many phases, including desire, excitement, orgasm, and resolution. Desire is showing or feeling an interest in sex. Excitement is the feeling of arousal. It can result from fantasy, erotic sights, sounds, scents, and tastes. The heart rate, pulse, and blood pressure will increase, as will respirations. Blood is sent to the genital area. The vagina becomes moist and enlarges in depth and width. The penis becomes erect and stiff. Orgasm is the sexual climax. The nervous system creates pleasurable sensation in the genital area, and the muscles around the genitals contract in a rhythmic manner. In men semen is ejaculated. In the resolution phase, the body returns to its previous unexcited state. Heart rate, pulse, and respirations slow down, blood drains from the genital area, and mental excitement subsides. In chronic illness, sexual problems may or may not occur. Problems may include low sexual desire, loss of vaginal mois-ture, painful intercourse, inability to reach orgasm, premature ejaculation, and inability to achieve or maintain an erection. Causes can include medications, surgical procedures, radiation, fatigue, loss of body image, loss of libido, and a fear of inability to perform (Arino-Norris, 1997; Dunn, 2000; Greif & Golden, 1994; Onel & Albertsen, 1999).

Patients with chronic illness do not stop being sexual simply because of the nature of their diagnosis. Sexuality remains an issue through the entirety of the life span. Although the expression of sexuality may take a back seat to the patient's diagnosis, it is never entirely forgotten. Feelings about sexuality influence the quality of life, self-image, and relationships. Sexuality is an aspect of the need for closeness, touch, pleasure, caring, and play. When sexual activity becomes difficult, impractical or impossible, such as during a period of severe illness or imminent death, expression of affection remains an important way to share intimacy.

Manifestations

- Avoidance of intimacy
- Preoccupation with sex
- Depression
- Increased somatic complaints
- Inability to achieve orgasm
- Psychosocial difficulty with intimate relationships

Strategies to Facilitate Individual Expression of Sexuality

A. Death is not imminent.
　1. Education
　　a) Provide information about the usual effects of the patient's diagnosis, medications, treatments, and surgery on sexuality.
　　b) Discuss high-risk versus low-risk sexual practices in regard to disease transmission (e.g., avoidance of the exchange of blood or body fluids).
　　c) Include information on contraception if appropriate.
　　d) Inform patients about alternatives to intercourse as an expression of sexuality (e.g., hugging, kissing, massage, caressing).
　　e) Discuss conservation of strength, rest periods, and preparation (Arino-Norris, 1997; Greif & Golden, 1994; Onel & Albertsen, 1999; Skolnick, 1999).
　2. Communication
　　a) Open communication (e.g., healthcare provider to patient, patient to partner) is essential for sexual health.
　　b) Embarrassment is often a barrier to be overcome.
　　c) Healthcare providers must take the lead by bringing up the subject for discussion.
　　　(1) Cultural and religious diversity must be acknowledged.
　　　(2) Lifestyle, gender, sexual orientation, marital status, and age all will play a part in communication.
　　　(3) Discussion of how specific diagnosis, treatment, or medications can affect sexuality should take place (Arino-Norris; Greif & Golden; Onel & Albertsen; Skolnick; Steinke, 2000).
　3. Lubrication ($)
　　a) For women experiencing a lack of vaginal moisture, a water-based gel, without perfumes or coloring, can be used. They are available over the counter.

b) Oil-based lubricants should be avoided because they can cause yeast infections in some women and are not compatible for use with latex condoms (Arino-Norris; Dunn, 2000; Greif & Golden).

4. Pain medications ($–$$)
   a) Pain may be nongenital because of surgery, for instance, or genital because of the narrowing of the vagina from radiation treatments to the area.
   b) When possible, pain medication should be taken approximately one hour prior to a sexual encounter to allow time for it to take effect.
   c) Narcotic or non-narcotic pain relievers can be used, depending upon the type, severity, and location of pain (Arino-Norris; Dunn; Muellar, 1997).

5. Positioning
   a) Use of a position that puts the least amount of pressure on the painful area is advised.
   b) Support of the painful area with pillows can assist in decreasing discomfort.
   c) For intercourse, recommend a position that puts the patient in control over movement (e.g., depth of thrust, speed) (Arino-Norris; Dunn; Muellar; Onel & Albertsen; Steinke).

6. Relaxation (0–$$)
   a) Once pain is felt during intercourse, the patient usually becomes tense awaiting another episode of pain.
   b) Patients may be nervous because of the length of time since their last sexual encounter and change that may have occurred since that time (e.g., surgical scars, hair loss, weight changes).
   c) Relaxation techniques include paced breathing, biofeedback, meditation, massage, visualization, or guided imagery. These can help the patient relax and avoid the pain associated with being tense.
   d) Kegel exercises can be practiced to help female patients become aware of their vaginal muscles and learn to relax them. Patients can practice Kegels by stopping the urine flow for a few seconds (tightening the muscles) and then relaxing. (Arino-Norris; Dunn; Greif & Golden; Onel & Albertsen).

7. Medication ($–$$$)
   a) Used to treat problems such as erectile dysfunction, vaginal dryness, and anxiety. Erectile dysfunction may be treated with sildenafil (Viagra®).
   b) Problems such as vaginal dryness may require hormone replacement therapy.
   c) Cost, dose, and interactions with other drugs or food will vary, and prescribing is individual to the patient and circumstance.
   d) Thorough education about the prescribed medication must take place and should include how and when to take the medication and side effects (Arino-Norris; Dunn; Onel & Albertsen).

8. Counseling/therapy ($$–$$$)
   a) Can occur in a sexual dysfunction clinic or in private practice.

b) Costs will vary greatly as will the number of visits needed. May involve learning new skills and practicing them with a partner.

c) A sex therapist should be a mental health professional (e.g., psychiatrist, social worker, psychologist) or a medical professional (e.g., physician, nurse) who is specially trained in treating sexual problems.

d) Other types of counseling or therapy can be helpful. Issues of depression, body image changes, social changes, and relationship alterations may require supportive counseling.

e) Support groups can be beneficial and are available in most communities (Arino-Norris; Dunn; Greif & Golden; Onel & Albertsen).

B. Death is imminent: Sexuality should be expressed at the comfort level of the patient and may take the form of hand-holding, a kiss, a look, a smile, or verbalization.

Patient Outcomes

A. Identifies sexual problems, dysfunction, or concerns

B. Attains satisfaction with self as a sexual being

C. Shares intimacy with partner at the level that is possible

Professional Competencies

A. A nonjudgmental approach to care is maintained.

B. Identification of sexual dysfunction and underlying cause(s) are identified early in the course of care.

C. The appropriateness of each intervention is determined by the patient with partner input.

D. Effectiveness of interventions is assessed and the treatment plan modified, as needed, for optimal outcome.

E. Sensitivity to cultural, religious, and sexual preference is maintained.

F. Sexual intimacy and expression are encouraged.

References

Arino-Norris, N. (1997). Sexual concerns after an MI. *American Journal of Nursing, 97,* 48–49.

Dunn, M. (2000). Sexual issues in older adults. *AIDS Patient Care and STDs, 14,* 67–69.

Greif, J., & Golden, B. (1994). *AIDS care at home.* New York: John Wiley & Sons.

Muellar, I. (1997). Common questions about sex and sexuality in elders. *American Journal of Nursing, 97,* 61–64.

Onel, E., & Albertsen, P. (1999). Management of impotence. *The Clinical Advisor, 1,* 27–37.

Skolnick, A. (1999). Talking to teens about sex. *Hippocrates, 1,* 25–29.

Steinke, E. (2000). Sexual counseling after myocardial infarction. *American Journal of Nursing, 100,* 38–43.

Skin Lesions

Debra E. Heidrich, RN, MSN, CHPN, AOCN®

Definitions

Pressure ulcers are wounds that involve cellular necrosis because of pressure or shearing force. Malignant cutaneous wounds are skin lesions that develop when malignant cells infiltrate the epithelium.

Pathophysiology/Etiology

Pressure ulcers are common at the end of life because of the effects of weakness, immobility, and inadequate nutrition. When soft tissue is compressed between a bony prominence and an external surface, the blood supply is disrupted. This results in ischemia, edema, and inflammation, followed by cell death (Agency for Healthcare Research and Quality [AHRQ], 1992; Hess, 1999).

Malignant cutaneous wounds occur when tumor cells infiltrate the epithelium as well as the lymph and blood vessels supporting the epithelium. Cell death occurs because of a lack of oxygen and nutrients when the blood flow is disrupted (Haisfield-Wolfe & Baxendale-Cox, 1999; Mortimer, 1998).
- Bleeding is common because of capillary rupture.
- Disruption of the lymph vessels can lead to significant drainage.
- Anaerobic organisms proliferate in necrotic tissue and cause foul-smelling odor.
- Aerobic organisms cause purulent discharge.

Manifestations

Skin ulcers are staged according to their color, size, appearance, and drainage. (Staging systems are described later in this section.) In addition, clinical manifestations may include
- Pain
- Infection

- Anemia
- Odor.

The distress and embarrassment from open, draining, and malodorous wounds also may lead to
- Self-concept disturbances
- Social isolation
- Anxiety or fear
- Depression.

Management

A. General measures
   1. Identify the stage of the lesion.
      a) Pressure ulcer staging (AHRQ, 1992)
         (1) Stage I: Nonblanchable erythema of intact skin
         (2) Stage II: Partial thickness skin loss involving the epidermis or dermis. These lesions appear as superficial abrasions, blisters, or shallow craters.
         (3) Stage III: Full thickness skin loss involving damage or necrosis of subcutaneous tissue. These lesions appear as deep craters and may or may not have undermining of adjacent tissues.
         (4) Stage IV: Full thickness skin loss with extensive destruction, tissue necrosis, or damage to muscle, bone, or supporting structures. These lesions appear as deep craters; undermining and sinus tracts are common.
      b) Malignant cutaneous wound staging (Haisfield-Wolfe & Baxendale-Cox, 1999)
         (1) Stage I: Closed, dry wound that is red/pink in color
         (2) Stage I–N: Wound that occasionally opens superficially to drain, then closes again. The wound color is red/pink and drainage may be clear or purulent. These wounds may be painful.
         (3) Stage II: Partial thickness skin loss involving dermal and epidermal tissue. The wound color is red/pink and drainage may be serosanguinous or sanguinous. These wounds may be painful and tend to be malodorous.
         (4) Stage III: Full thickness skin loss involving subcutaneous tissue. The wound color may be red/pink or yellow, and drainage is purulent or serosanguinous. These wounds are most likely painful and tend to be malodorous.
         (5) Stage IV: Full thickness skin loss with invasion into deep anatomic tissues and structures. Tunneling is often present. The wound color may be red/pink or yellow, and drainage is serosanguinous, sanguinous, or purulent. Pain is likely, and the wound tends to be malodorous.

2. Prevent pressure ulcers.
   a) Keep skin clean and dry.
   b) Prevent friction and shear injuries.
      (1) Use care with patient transfers and turning, using lift pads or turning sheets.
      (2) Reduce friction on heels and elbows by using lubricants, thin film dressings, or protectors.
   c) Encourage mobility and range-of-motion exercises based on an individual's ability to tolerate these activities.
   d) Reduce pressure on tissues.
      (1) Turn and reposition at least every two hours.
      (2) Avoid positioning on trochanter.
      (3) Use supports, such as wedges, pillows, and heel supports.
      (4) Consider using specialty mattresses, especially for those at greatest risk ($$$) (AHRQ; Hess, 1999).
      (5) Avoid massage over bony prominences (AHRQ).

B. Death is not imminent.
   1. Treat malignant cutaneous wounds.
      a) Use radiation therapy or chemotherapy ($$$) for localized lesions. This may decrease bleeding, drainage, and pain (Mortimer, 1998).
      b) Hormonal manipulation ($$–$$$)—May be helpful for lesions associated with breast cancer (Waller & Caroline, 2000)
   2. Care for and dress the ulcer appropriately.
      a) Irrigation ($)
         (1) No sign of infection—Flush with normal saline or water, using a bulb syringe or gravity drip through IV tubing.
         (2) Infected or foul-smelling wounds—Cleanse with one of the following agents and then rinse with normal saline or water. Discontinue use of these agents as soon as infection is adequately treated, as these solutions are toxic to fibroblasts and will inhibit wound healing (Hess, 1999).
            (a) Acetic acid solution ($) (equal parts vinegar and water) for *Pseudomonas* infection
            (b) Hydrogen peroxide ($) for mechanical cleansing of crusted exudates
            (c) Povidone iodine ($) for broad-spectrum antimicrobial cleansing
            (d) Sodium hypochlorite ($) (1 part household bleach to 9 parts water) (Dakin's solution) for staphylococcal and streptococcal infections
      b) Debridement
         (1) Usually appropriate in the palliative care setting unless necrotic tissue in the ulcer is a source of infection or pain
         (2) Use of enzymatic debriding agents ($$$), such as collagenase (Santyl®), fibrinolysin (Elase®), or papain urea (Accuzyme®); pro-

motion of autolytic debridement using transparent film, hydrocolloid, or semipermeable urethane foam; or hydrogel dressings ($$) are the preferred methods of debridement in the palliative setting (Hess, 1999; Waller & Caroline).

c) Clean skin around wound with saline or water.

d) Pack deep wounds with wound pastes, granules, powders, beads, or gels ($$–$$$). These promote a moist healing environment, promote autolytic debridement, absorb exudates, and promote comfort (Hess).

e) Cover with a dressing that promotes a moist healing environment.
   (1) Stage I–II: Polyurethane transparent film dressings ($$)
   (2) Stage II–III: Hydrocolloid dressings ($$)
   (3) Use an absorbent dressing for significant exudate ($$).
   (4) If drainage exceeds 50 ml/day, consider using a wound-drainage bag to collect exudate, decrease number of dressing changes required, control odor, and protect surrounding skin (Hess).

f) Control bleeding.
   (1) Apply pressure to visible bleeding vessels if underlying structures can tolerate the pressure.
   (2) Apply silver nitrate sticks ($$) to pinpoint capillary oozing. Note that this may cause pain and patient should be medicated appropriately.
   (3) Apply gauze soaked in 1:1000 epinephrine ($$) (Waller & Caroline).
   (4) Use a coagulant dressing, such as absorbable gelatin (Gelfoam®) ($$).
   (5) Consider radiation therapy ($$$$) (Mortimer).

g) Control odor. No studies are available to compare the benefits and burdens of the following interventions.
   (1) Topical metronidazole (Flagyl®) gel, 0.75%–0.80% ($$) or irrigation with parenteral metronidazole solution (Finlay, Bowszyc, Ramlau, & Gwiezdzinski, 1996). Chlorophyll-containing ointments ($$) applied to wound or chlorophyll tablets taken po.
   (2) Odor-filtering dressings that have a carbon or charcoal layer ($$).
   (3) Active culture plain yogurt applied to the wound may help to eliminate anaerobic organisms, but application is messy and time-consuming ($ for yogurt; $$ for caregiver time).
   (4) Deodorizers may mask odors. Some people may find the scent of the deodorizer offensive.
      (a) Dressing deodorizers ($$) (Banish®, Hexon®) may be used sparingly on dressings.
      (b) Commercial room deodorizers, scented candles, or scented oils ($) may be used in the room.

h) Assess severity of pain and treat appropriately. This may require topical or systemic analgesics.

C. Death is imminent.

1. Continue an appropriate positioning and turning schedule to prevent the pain of tissue ischemia.
   a) Be sure to use good technique, ideally with two persons, to prevent discomfort.
   b) Use nursing judgment to balance any discomfort associated with turning against potential discomfort of tissue ischemia.
   c) Premedicate for turning, if needed.
2. Continue to manage drainage, odor, and pain related to the ulcer.

Patient Outcomes

A. Prevention of pressure ulcers whenever possible

B. Healing of pressure ulcers

C. Absence of infection related to skin lesions whenever possible

D. Relief of physical discomfort and prevention of complications associated with skin lesions

Professional Competencies

A. Risk for pressure ulcers is identified.

B. Interventions to prevent/minimize pressure ulcers are selected based on the condition of the patient and the abilities of caregivers.

C. Appropriate cleansing agents and dressings are selected based on the type of wound, the presence of infection or odor, and the presence of exudate or drainage.

D. Caregivers are taught appropriate skin care and wound care interventions, based on patient need and caregiver abilities.

References

Agency for Healthcare Research and Quality. (1992). *Pressure ulcers in adults: Prediction and prevention. Clinical practice guideline no. 3.* Rockville, MD: Author.

Finlay, I.G., Bowszyc, J., Ramlau, C., & Gwiezdzinski, Z. (1996). The effect of topical 0.75% metronidazole gel on malodorous cutaneous ulcers. *Journal of Pain and Symptom Management, 22,* 158–162.

Haisfield-Wolfe, M.E., & Baxendale-Cox, L.M. (1999). Staging of malignant cutaneous wounds: A pilot study. *Oncology Nursing Forum, 26,* 1055–1064.

Hess, C.T. (1999). *Clinical guide: Wound care* (3rd ed.). Springhouse, PA: Springhouse.

Mortimer, P.S. (1998). Management of skin problems: Medical aspects. In D. Doyle, G.W.C. Hanks, & N. MacDonald (Eds.), *Oxford textbook of palliative medicine* (2nd ed.) (pp. 617–627). New York: Oxford University Press.

Waller, A., & Caroline, N.L. (2000). *Handbook of palliative care in cancer.* Boston: Butterworth-Heinemann.

Spirituality

Rev. James M. Deshotels, SJ, APRN

Definition

Spirituality has many definitions, reflecting the mystery and ineffability of human nature and spiritual experience. Amenta (1997) offered a particularly succinct definition: "The spiritual realm can be broadly defined as the life force springing from the unknown that pervades each person's entire being." This concept of human spirit embraces and encompasses all other aspects of human personality and need. The spiritual or existential needs of the dying are similar to those that occur throughout the life span and are intimately connected. These include the need for affiliation; the need to love and be loved; interaction at one's level of physical, mental, psychologic, and spiritual capability; a sense of purpose and hope; and a sense of making a contribution, however limited, to the lives of others (Amenta; Taylor, Amenta, & Highfield, 1995).

Specific Issues Related to Palliative Care
Spiritual Needs Are as Unique and Varied as Individuals and Families

Appropriate strategies for assessment and intervention will reflect the varied temperaments, experience, clinical wisdom, and human genius of the interdisciplinary healthcare team, patient, and family. Strategies beneficial to one family unit may well be inappropriate for others, even when they have similar diagnoses and demographics.

Ruling Out Physical Causes of Restlessness, Anxiety, or Discomfort

Unresolved spiritual or psychosocial issues should not be confused with physical symptoms. In assessments, the interdisciplinary team should include or collaborate with appropriate clergy, members of religious orders, parish nurses (a relatively new specialty), and lay congregational health ministers, as well as psychiatry, psychology, and social services professionals.

Manifestations of Spiritual Distress

- Grieving for loss of life, function, abilities, loved ones
- Expressions of fear
- Anxiety and fear related to diagnosis, treatment, pain, the future, the needs and future of significant others, the unknown, or dying
- Expressions of anger, whether nonspecific or directed at God, other people, or self
- Depression, sadness, grief, hopelessness, or despair
- Guilt, anger, sorrow about past actions, decisions, life choices, or relationships
- Difficulties in relating to caregivers and significant others because of physical limitations, distance, or economics
- Social withdrawal, restlessness, and sleeplessness
- Acting out

Indications of Spiritual Coping

- Honest requests to talk about psychosocial, spiritual, or religious matters or to see clergy or mental healthcare professionals
- Questions about death (e.g., what dying would be like, how it might be carried out with dignity, living wills, practitioners' beliefs about life after death)
- Questions or statements reflecting a search for meaning in life or terminal illness
- Religious articles and books at the bedside
- References to prayer, God, or faith

(Rakel & Storey, 1993; Stepnick & Perry, 1992; Taylor et al., 1995)

Strategies to Facilitate Individual Spirituality

A. Take a holistic approach to care.
  1. The whole patient is cared for by an interdisciplinary approach. The interdisciplinary team ideally includes a spiritual care coordinator (as in hospice care (Beresford, 1997).
  2. The physiologic, social, or economic stressors on the spiritual and psychosocial well-being should not be ignored.
  3. Physical modalities—such as heat, cold, positioning, therapeutic touch, and massage—can potentiate cognitive and pharmacologic interventions as well as strengthen the human bonds between patients and caregivers.
  4. The importance of the basic techniques of therapeutic listening and conversation should not be underestimated.

B. Provide opportunities for open, nonjudgmental discussion (Stanhope & Knollmueller, 1996; Stepnick & Perry, 1992; Taylor et al., 1995).

1. Encourage patients and their families to talk about the losses they already have experienced, are currently experiencing, and those they anticipate. If appropriate, encourage patients to talk about how their faith gives them strength to cope with difficulties.
2. Acknowledge that patients and significant others will vary in their ability to assimilate changes and that a range of reactions and coping strategies is normal.
3. Consider ways that the patient can remain involved with family life (prevent social death).
4. Help sort out family members' expectations with regard to the dying member, each other, and themselves.
5. Legitimize respite time and help patients and families incorporate it from the outset.
6. Help patients and family members understand the dynamics of the situation that contribute to their complex and ambivalent feelings.
7. Use community resources to support the family when their resources are insufficient.
8. Appreciate that helping does not always entail finding an answer or a specific solution.
9. Normalize the transition, and help patients and family members understand the dynamics associated with the paradoxes they face (keep on living while preparing for death).
10. Provide a sounding board for sorting out thoughts and feelings.
11. Be aware of your own comfort level in dealing with situations that are paradoxical and arouse ambivalent feelings.
12. Do not force discussion on difficult topics, but appraise whether the hesitation comes from within you or the family.
13. Encourage life review and recognize that this may include regrets and pain as well as pleasant memories.
14. Help patients and families to include children in the process rather than exclude them.
15. Affirm patients and families for their ability to manage and create goodness amid tragedy.

Patient Outcomes

A. Experiences fulfillment in whatever level of spirituality is desired

B. Experiences a feeling of being at peace

C. Experiences freedom to express spiritual issues without restrictions

Professional Competencies

A. Demonstrate therapeutic use of self.

B. Listen and demonstrate concern for the patient and his or her loved ones.

C. Respect individual worldviews and awareness of differences.

D. Understand one's own spirituality and spiritual needs.

E. Seek spiritual support, counseling, or supervision when encountering difficult situations.

(Stanhope & Knollmueller, 1996; Stepnick & Perry, 1992; Taylor et al., 1995)

References

Amenta, M. (1997). Editorial. *International Journal of Palliative Nursing, 3,* 1.

Beresford, L. (1997). The updated book on prayer: Spiritual care strives to hold its place on the hospice team. *Hospice, 22,* 22–26.

Rakel, R.E., & Storey, P. (1993). Care of the dying patient. In R. Rakel (Ed.), *Essentials of family practice* (pp. 68–81). Philadelphia: W.B. Saunders.

Stanhope, M., & Knollmueller, R.N. (1996). *Handbook of community and home health nursing* (2nd ed.). St. Louis, MO: Mosby.

Stepnick, A., & Perry, T. (1992). Preventing spiritual distress in the dying client. *Journal of Psychosocial Nursing, 30,* 17–24.

Taylor, E.J., Amenta, M., & Highfield, M. (1995). Spiritual care practices of oncology nurses. *Oncology Nursing Forum, 22,* 31–39.

Terminal Sedation

Helen K. McHale, MSN, RN, CHPN

Definition

Terminal sedation is defined as a medical procedure used to palliate end-stage symptoms refractory to sequentially trialed standardized interventions. Terminal sedation is accomplished by intentionally dimming the patient's consciousness through pharmaceutical interventions. Sedation may be intermittent or continuous and is distinguished from active euthanasia by using medication to the point of unconsciousness, not death. The ethical principle of "double effect" holds that aggressive symptom management resulting in death is not euthanasia as long as the intent is to relieve symptoms and provide comfort (Martinez & Groth, 2000; Morita, Tsunoda, Inoue, & Chihara, 2000).

Pathophysiology/Etiology

Despite standardized pain and symptom management practices, occasional situations occur when the patient's illness produces unrelenting tenacious, intractable pain or discomfort. The change in symptoms suddenly may emerge and rapidly escalate to literally unbearable proportions. Patients at risk for the development of excruciating pain include those who have bony metastases, cranial cancers, head and neck cancers, neuropathic pain, extremely rapid tumor growth, past history of alcoholism, and preexisting psychiatric problems. Other unrelieved symptoms despite aggressive management can include dyspnea, delirium, and restlessness.

Additional factors that may require sedation include the withholding or withdrawing of life support, violent vomiting, massive bleeding, or unrelenting seizures (Coyle & Truog, 1994).

Manifestations

The following indicate the potential need for terminal sedation.
• Intolerable pain in the last 48 hours

- Uncontrolled dyspnea
- Delirium
- Terminal restlessness/agitation
- Status epilepticus
- Any intractable symptoms that become unbearable for the patient
- Hemorrhaging

Management

A. General
1. Sedation should be administered only after discussing with the patient and his or her support system and receiving consent to use this intervention as a palliative measure to relieve intractable symptoms.
2. Pharmaceutical sedation should be administered at the onset of a disturbing symptom.
3. Medication is administered until the patient reaches the state of sedation and appears comfortable and no longer bothered by his or her symptoms.
4. Respite and subsequent sedation can be individualized by decreasing, discontinuing, or restarting medication. Intermittent sedation provides essential rest for the patient.
5. Continuous sedation is reserved for unrelenting physical or emotional suffering, prevention of suicide, and withholding or withdrawing of life support. The medication level in continuous sedation is titrated with adjustments to maintain a somnolent state.

B. Death is imminent.
1. All treatable causes and conceivable interventions for symptom control have been exhausted.
2. Professional staff providing patient care understands the intent is not to hasten death but to minimize discomfort until natural death occurs.
3. A do not resuscitate order must be in effect. At no time should the decision for sedation be made without the consent of the patient or the proxy.
4. Once a decision for sedation is made, initiation is swift. Titration continues until relief, subanesthesia, or somnolence occurs.
5. The patient receives continuous evaluation for sedation effectiveness and is continually assessed and treated for other symptoms: pain, dyspnea and secretions, vomiting, seizures, or bleeding.
6. Hydrating oral care is provided every 20–30 minutes as needed. The patient is turned and positioned every two to three hours and as needed.
7. The patient is never left alone while sedated and is calmly touched and spoken to during care.

C. Medications (Twycross & Lichter, 1998)
1. The sedation usually demands alternate routes for medications, but administration does not need to be technical.

2. Most of these medications can be given rectally, sublingually (buccal or gingival), or subcutaneously, either by infusion or injection.
3. Patients must continue to receive opiates and adjuvant analgesics.
4. Intermittent or continuous sedation
    a) Upward titration of opioid medication may provide sedating relief. If not, consider adding an antianxiety agent, such as
        (1) Diazepam (Valium®) ($)—5–20 mg titrated as needed or as an hourly drip (topical, sl, pr, or IV)
        (2) Lorazepam (Ativan®) ($)—considered five times stronger than diazepam; 1 mg titrated as needed (topical, sl, pr, or IV).
    b) If the above is not helpful, continue opiate medication and consider changing to
        (1) Midazolam (Versed®) ($$)—2–6 mg/hour (sq or IV drip)
        (2) Triazolam (Halcion®) ($)—0.25 mg several times/day (sl or pr).
    c) For a confused or agitated patient, continue opiate and start with
        (1) Chlorpromazine (Thorazine®) ($)—100–200 mg, titrate as needed up to 800 mg (sl, pr, sq, or IM)
        (2) Droperidol (Inapsine®) ($)—1.25–2.5 mg every 2–4 hours (IM or IV).
    d) To keep the patient sedated, continue opiate and use
        (1) Diazepam ($)—5–20 mg pr immediately and every 6–8 hours
        (2) Midazolam ($$)—5–20 mg immediately and 60 mg sq over 24 hours by continuous infusion, titrating to achieve control.
    e) If the previous two medications fail, continue opiate and use phenobarbital ($)—200 mg sq infusion immediately and 600–1,200 mg/24 hours continuous sq infusion.
    f) For extrapyramidal signs and symptoms, add diphenhydramine (Benadryl®) ($)—50 mg every 6 hours as needed (sl, pr, IM, or IV).
    g) To control muscle twitching or focal seizures that accompany sedation (very distressing for relatives)
        (1) Diazepam ($)—10 mg q 4–6 hours (sl, pr, IM, or IV).
        (2) Clonazepam (Klonopin®) ($)—0.5–2 mg bid–tid (sl, pr, or IV)
        (3) Phenobarbital ($)—10–20 mg bid–qid (sl, pr, or sq) (Coluzzi, Volker, & Miaskowski, 1996; Twycross & Lichter; Wrede-Seaman, 1999).

Patient Outcomes

A. Pain and symptom reduction with accompanied comfort

B. Understanding that terminal sedation is aggressive management for intractable pain and symptoms

C. Understanding that the eventual outcome of this intervention is death

Professional Competencies

A. Identify that the treatment of pain and suffering is the highest priority in caring for the terminally ill.

B. Recognize that treatment of pain and suffering by administering both analgesics and sedatives is noncontroversial.

C. Demonstrate appropriate selection, use, and titration of sedating medications.

References

Coluzzi, P.H., Volker, B., & Miaskowski, C. (Eds.). (1996). *Comprehensive pain management in terminal illness.* Sacramento, CA: California State Hospice Association.

Coyle, N., & Truog, R.D. (1994). Healthcare ethics forum '94: Pain management and sedation in the terminally ill. *AACN Clinical Issues, 5,* 360–365.

Martinez, J., & Groth, L. (2000). Terminal sedation in the home. *Journal of Hospice and Palliative Nursing, 2,* 31–34.

Morita, T., Tsunoda, J., Inoue, S., & Chihara, S. (2000). Terminal sedation for existential distress. *American Journal of Hospice and Palliative Care, 17,* 189–195.

Twycross, R.G., & Lichter, I. (1998). The terminal phase. In D. Doyle, G.W.C. Hanks, & N. MacDonald (Eds.), *Oxford textbook of palliative medicine* (2nd ed.) (pp. 977–992). New York: Oxford University Press.

Wrede-Seaman, L. (1999). *Symptom management algorithms: A handbook for palliative care.* Yakima, WA: Intellicard.

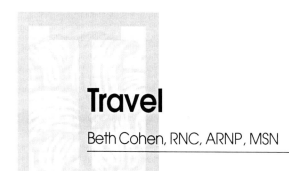

Travel

Beth Cohen, RNC, ARNP, MSN

The ability to travel can have a significant impact on quality of life for the individual with advanced disease. The goal of travel preparations for patients with advanced disease is to safeguard against possible problems that may arise as part of the travel experience.

Specific Issues Related to Palliative Care

- Physical discomfort
- Potential incontinence
- Pain
- Fatigue

Measures to Facilitate Travel

A. Death is not imminent.
   1. Health history
      a) Can be obtained from the patient's healthcare provider and should be with the patient and easily accessible during travel.
      b) Should include all relevant information, including current medications, allergies, and treatments.
      c) Travel companions should have access to it.
      d) Health history should be provided to the healthcare professional in charge of the patient's care, should the need arise, while traveling (Greif & Golden, 1994).
   2. Advance directive
      a) Must be with the patient at all times, and traveling companions should know where to find it.
      b) Included are documents designating healthcare surrogate and powers of attorney

    c) Healthcare providers will need to have a copy in the event the patient requires treatment while traveling (Greif & Golden).

3. Medication

    a) Patient should take along adequate amounts of medication in case plans change.

    b) Extra prescriptions should be obtained and packed in case of lost medication.

    c) Medication should be hand-carried when traveling, not packed in a suitcase to be loaded onto a plane or ship.

    d) Water also should be carried so the patient can take medication whenever needed (Greif & Golden).

4. Comfort: A patient should

    a) Anticipate the need for frequent rest periods.

    b) Stretch legs, use the bathroom, take medication, and snack

    c) Anticipate possible motion sickness. Medication may be prescribed as needed.

    d) Consider bringing a pillow for help with positioning.

    e) Dress appropriately and carry a sweater to adapt to temperature changes.

    f) Carry water to drink to prevent dehydration and facilitate the taking of medications.

    g) When possible, request ground-floor hotel rooms or choose hotels with elevators.

    h) Take advantage of privileges afforded to those traveling while ill, such as use of wheelchairs at airports, early boarding, and special meals.

    i) Bring needed medical equipment—such as toilet extender, adult diapers, walker, and cane—as they usually are not available at hotels or on planes (Greif & Golden).

    j) Carry a letter from the healthcare provider explaining the need to carry needles and syringes if injectable medications are being used.

5. Transportation

    a) Ambulance services can be used to transport patients from one place to another for a fee.

    b) This usually will not be covered by insurance unless used as transport to/from a medical facility (Greif & Golden).

B. Death is imminent.

1. Travel to the place where the patient would like to spend his or her last hours (usually home) should be by ambulance, and an acceptable form of a do not resuscitate order should accompany the patient.

2. Laws vary, including the need to have a different do not resuscitate form for inpatient and outpatient settings.

3. A significant other should travel with the patient whenever possible (Greif & Golden, 1994).

Patient Outcomes

A. Travel is planned with realistic expectations.

B. Ability to travel to desired location is achieved.

C. Comfort is maintained during travel.

D. Access to health care is maintained during the travel experience.

Professional Competencies

A. Appropriateness of travel is evaluated; problems are anticipated and solutions planned.

B. Arrangements are made to ensure continuity of care.

C. Effectiveness of interventions is evaluated, and plan is modified for optimal outcome.

D. Communication between healthcare providers is maintained to provide optimal quality of patient care.

Reference

Greif, J., & Golden, B.A. (1994). *AIDS care at home.* New York: John Wiley & Sons.

Urinary Elimination

Peg Esper, MSN, RN, CS, AOCN®

Definition

Urinary elimination is the process by which the body rids itself of waste products via the kidneys and bladder.

Pathophysiology/Etiology

The inability to void without difficulty and with control is a frequent source of frustration and anxiety for the patient with an advanced illness. Difficulties with urine elimination can be related to a number of clinical problems, including obstruction by tumor (e.g., prostate cancer, renal cancer, bladder cancer); altered renal function secondary to the disease process; or medications, including analgesics and anticholinergics. Inadequate urination also may be caused by impaired function of alternative urinary elimination devices. Diminished urination also is a natural process at the end of life (Kemp, 1999).

Manifestations

- Decreased or absent urinary output
- Hematuria or clots in urine
- Palpable bladder
- Inability to control voiding
- Lower abdominal discomfort
- Flank pain
- Straining to void

Management

A. General measures
   1. Identify potential reasons for the inability to void (i.e., problems with urine production or urine passage).

2. Evaluate the need for catheterization.
3. Evaluate the current medication profile for drugs that may interfere with the normal urinary process.
4. Evaluate adequacy of hydration/fluid intake and encourage the intake of fluids as appropriate.

B. Death is not imminent.
  1. Obstruction (Esper & Redman, 1999; Regnard & Tempest, 1998)
     a) Determine feasibility of intermittent self-catheterization (ISC) or an indwelling Foley catheter if needed for urinary patency ($).
     b) Evaluate need for percutaneous nephrostomy tube insertion ($$$).
     c) Consider the need for intermittent or continuous irrigation if clots are occluding the Foley catheter ($$).
        (1) Irrigate with normal saline.
        (2) For bleeding, instill 50 ml 1% alum solution for 30 minutes.
     d) Evaluate for obstruction of other urinary elimination devices.
     e) Evaluate need for maintenance antibiotic therapy when indwelling devices are used, to help prevent infection/sepsis.
     f) Evaluate need for embolization of tumor obstructing bladder neck ($$$).
  2. Incontinence (Kemp, 1999)
     a) Determine need for indwelling Foley catheter versus ISC based on patient and family preferences ($).
     b) Take measures to protect skin from breakdown ($).
     c) Consider use of antispasmodics/anticholinergics ($–$$)—oxybutynin hydrochloride (Ditropan®) 5 mg po bid–qid.

C. Death is imminent.
  1. A gradual decline in the filtering function of the kidneys is part of the terminal process.
  2. At this time, comfort is a priority, and use of a Foley catheter may be desirous to prevent incontinence of urine requiring frequent bed changes and patient movement.
  3. Evaluate caregiver preferences.

Patient Outcomes

A. Optimal urinary elimination

B. Prevention of skin breakdown

Professional Competencies

A. Recognize the potential etiologies associated with an alteration in urinary elimination.

B. Institute measures to improve/maintain optimal urinary elimination.

C. Recognize priority of comfort when death is imminent.

D. Evaluate patient and caregiver wishes related to possible interventions.

References

Esper, P., & Redman, B. (1999). Supportive care, pain management and quality of life in advanced prostate cancer. *Urologic Clinics of North America, 26,* 375–390.

Kemp, C. (1999). *Terminal illness* (2nd ed.). Philadelphia: J.B. Lippincott.

Regnard, C., & Tempest, S. (1998). *A guide to symptom relief in advanced disease.* Hale, England: Hochland & Hochland.

Xerostomia

Peg Esper, MSN, RN, CS, AOCN®

Definition

Xerostomia is dryness of the mouth that can range from mild to severe. A majority of terminally ill patients are affected with this problem.

Pathophysiology/Etiology

Saliva is an essential lubricant for the oral cavity. Xerostomia can be seen anytime individuals have had disruption of normal salivary flow/production. Contributing factors include radiation to the head and neck area, head and neck surgery resulting in damage or the removal of salivary glands, Sjögren's syndrome, certain medications (e.g., anticholinergics, antihistamines, morphine, tricyclic antidepressants), and infections. Excessive dryness of the mouth, based on the severity of xerostomia experienced, can affect the individual's ability to eat, swallow, speak, taste, and sleep (Davies, 1997; Holmes, 1998; Iwamoto, 1999).

Manifestations

- Dysphagia
- Dysphonia
- Decreased taste sensation
- Decreased ability to chew
- Soreness of mouth
- Thickened or absent saliva

Management

A. Frequent oral rinses and fastidious oral hygiene

B. Soft, moist foods (e.g., use of sauces, gravies)

C. Sucking on hard, sour candy

D. Use of a spray bottle to mist the oral cavity

E. Artificial saliva products ($)

F. Chewing gum

G. Canola oil in the mouth at bedtime

H. Pilocarpine (Salagen®) tablets (5 mg po tid) ($)

I. Antifungal agents to treat oral infections (nystatin [Mycostatin®], fluconazole [Diflucan®]) ($–$$)

J. Acupuncture ($$)

K. Sweet, hard candies and lemon-glycerin swabs should be avoided, as they increase dryness and thickness of saliva.
(Davies, 1997; Holmes, 1998; Iwamoto, 1999; Rydholm, 1999)

Patient Outcomes

A. Adequate lubrication of the oral cavity

B. Optimal comfort

Professional Competencies

A. Identify those factors that may lead to the development of xerostomia.

B. Institute measures to decrease the manifestations of xerostomia and modify the treatment plan as appropriate.

C. Intact oral mucosa is maintained.

References

Davies, A. (1997). The management of xerostomia: A review. *European Journal of Cancer Care, 6,* 209–214.

Holmes, S. (1998). Xerostomia: Aetiology and management in cancer patients. *Supportive Care in Cancer, 6,* 348–355.

Iwamoto, R. (1999). Xerostomia. In C. Yarbro, M. Frogge, & M. Goodman (Eds.), *Cancer symptom management* (pp. 264–272). Boston: Jones and Bartlett.

Rydholm, M. (1999). Acupuncture for patients in hospital-based home care suffering from xerostomia. *Journal of Palliative Care, 15,* 20–23.

Zoster

Peg Esper, MSN, RN, CS, AOCN®

Definition

Zoster (*Varicella zoster* virus [VZV], shingles) is a viral infection resulting from reactivation of the latent VZV in the dorsal root ganglia. Considerable morbidity can result when the virus becomes disseminated outside of its original dermatome. Both cutaneous and visceral dissemination are possible (Freifeld, Walsh, & Pizzo, 1999).

Pathophysiology/Etiology

Reactivation of the VZV is a common complication in terminally ill individuals as a result of their increased immunosuppression. Mortality rates as high as 10% have been reported and are frequently linked to the development of VZV pneumonia or central nervous system invasion leading to encephalitis (Freifeld et al., 1999).

Manifestations

*   Vesicular lesions along a dermatome
*   Intense neuropathic-like pain
*   Abdominal discomfort
*   Symptoms related to encephalitis

Management

A. Death is not imminent (Freifeld et al., 1999; Whitmore, 1999).
    1. Antivirals
        a) Acyclovir (Zovirax®) ($$)—800 mg every 4 hours (five times daily) orally for 7–10 days

    b) Famciclovir (Famvir®) ($$)—500 mg orally every 8 hours for 7 days

    c) Valacyclovir (Valtrex®) ($$)—1 g orally every 8 hours for 7 days

  2. Analgesics

    a) Topical capsaicin (Zostrix®) ($)—cream applied four times daily (for control of postherpetic neuralgia)

    b) See Pain and Appendix A.

  3. Meticulous oral care: For herpes zoster affecting the oral region

B. Death is imminent.

  1. Priority is given to keeping the individual comfortable.

  2. The use of antivirals at this time is of little value.

Patient Outcomes

A. Symptoms associated with the VZV infection are controlled.

B. Lesions on skin/mucous membrane are healed/show signs of healing.

Professional Competencies

A. Identify VZV lesions.

B. Recognize symptoms of dissemination of the virus.

C. Institute measures to decrease symptoms from acute infection.

D. Institute measures to decrease neuropathic pain.

E. Evaluate patient response and modify treatment plan as appropriate.

References

Freifeld, A., Walsh, T., & Pizzo, P. (1999). Infections in the cancer patient. In V.T. Devita, S. Hellman, & S.A. Rosenberg (Eds.), *Cancer: Principles and practice of oncology* (pp. 2659–2704). Philadelphia: Lippincott-Raven.

Whitmore, S.E. (1999). Common problems of the skin. In L.R. Barker, J.R. Burton, & P.D. Zieve (Eds.), *Principles of ambulatory medicine* (pp. 1499–1539). Baltimore: Williams & Wilkins.

Appendix A
Management of Neuropathic Pain

Marco Pappagallo, MD, E. Duke Dickerson, MSc, PhD,
James Varga, RPh, MBA, Joshua M. Cox, RPh,
Costantino Benedetti, MD, and Mellar Davis, MD,
FCCP

Pharmacologic Agents With Some Established Efficacy for Neuropathic Pain

Anticonvulsant Drugs

Anticonvulsant drugs (ACDs) are becoming the most promising agents for the management of neuropathic pain. Gabapentin (Neurontin®) has been shown to be effective for the treatment of postherpetic neuralgia (i.e., a neuropathic state characterized by allodynia and spontaneous burning pain) and painful diabetic neuropathy (i.e., a state characterized predominantly by spontaneous burning pain) (Baconja et al., 1998; Rowbotham, Harden, Stacey, Bernstein, & Magnus-Miller, 1998).

Gabapentin acts on neither gamma-aminobutyric acid (GABA) receptors nor sodium channels, and its analgesic mechanism of action is unclear. Trigeminal neuralgia (i.e., a neuropathic condition characterized by brief, excruciating lancinating facial pains) responds well to carbamazepine (Tegretol®), while another ACD, lamotrigine (Lamictal®), has shown some efficacy for carbamazepine-resistant trigeminal neuralgia (Zakrzewska, Chaudhry, Nurmikko, Patton, & Mullens, 1997). Several new ACDs (levetiracetam [Keppra™], zonisamide [Zonegran®], oxcarbazepine [Trileptal®], and tiagabine [Gabitril®]) have become available for medical use in the United States. Some of these agents may have potential analgesic properties. For example, preliminary data suggest that the ACD zonisamide, a blocker of sodium and T-type calcium channels, may have an antineuropathic analgesic effect (Tomlinson, Malcangio, Patel, Meyer, & Chen, 1999).

Opiates

Opiates are currently the most potent and effective analgesics used to treat acute and chronic painful states, and, as such, they have been prescribed to patients suffering from intractable pain states. Morphine, a mu agonist, represents the mainstay for the treatment of moderate to severe nociceptive cancer pain

(Pappagallo, 1999; Portenoy, 1996). Evidence from recent controlled trials also has shown the efficacy of opiate analgesics in the treatment of neuropathic pain (Suzuki, Chapman, & Dickenson, 1999). Pure opiate agonists, morphine, fentanyl, methadone, levorphanol, oxycodone, hydromorphone, and hydrocodone, are the mainstay of opiate therapy. The treatment of chronic pain should rely on the use of long-acting agents (e.g., methadone, levorphanol) or controlled-release preparations of morphine, fentanyl, oxycodone, and hydromorphone. Among the pure opiate agonists, methadone has peculiar properties—an intrinsic N-methyl-D-aspartate receptor antagonistic effect, which may add adjuvant analgesia in neuropathic pain.

Unlike anti-inflammatory drugs, opiate agonists have no analgesic "ceiling dose" and do not cause direct organ damage. Except for constipation, tolerance occurs for most of the opiate-related side effects (e.g., nausea, vomiting, respiratory depression, drowsiness). *Opiate titration* and *opiate rotation* are essential concepts in the management of neuropathic pain. To determine adequate opiate responsiveness, a careful and persistent titration of the opiate is needed (Pappagallo, 1999). However, opiate-related side effects and the degrees of analgesia and tolerance are extremely variable among patients receiving these medications. Neuropathic pain may respond well to morphine, but in some patients, it responds only to methadone and in others to fentanyl (Portenoy, 1996). Trials of different opiates (i.e., opiate rotation) have strongly been encouraged, especially when, during the initial drug trial, severe pain persists or side effects become intolerable.

Tricyclic Antidepressants

Tricyclic antidepressants (TCAs), such as amitriptyline (Elavil®), nortriptyline (Pamelor®), and desipramine (Norpramin®), have established efficacy for neuropathic pain. They have been used successfully for painful diabetic neuropathy and postherpetic neuralgia. TCAs may provide pain relief in patients who are not depressed who are affected by neuropathic pain. TCAs have frequent adverse effects to which tolerance develops poorly. The side effects include cardiotoxicity, confusion, urinary retention, orthostatic hypotension, nightmares, weight gain, drowsiness, dry mouth, and constipation.

Venlafaxine (Effexor®) is a newer antidepressant that lacks the anticholinergic and antihistamine effects of the TCAs. Venlafaxine appears to possess an analgesic mechanism of action, with similar TCA-like beneficial properties but fewer side effects (Lang, Hord, & Denson, 1996; Schreiber, Backer, & Pick, 1999). Selective serotonin reuptake inhibitors such as paroxetine (Paxil®) and fluoxetine (Prozac®) are effective antidepressants but have not been as efficacious as TCAs (Max et al., 1992).

Local and Topical Analgesics

Local anesthetics, such as intravenous lidocaine and oral mexiletine (Mexitil®), have been used in patients with neuropathic pain (Wallace, 2000). The antiarrhythmic local anesthetic mexiletine is a sodium channel blocker with analgesic properties for neuropathic pain similar to those of some ACDs (e.g., lamotrigine, carbamazepine). Mexiletine is contraindicated in the presence of second- and third-degree atrium-ventricular conduction blocks. Also, the incidence of gastrointestinal side effects (e.g., diarrhea, nausea) is quite high in patients taking mexiletine. Intravenous lidocaine has been shown to decrease pain in patients with postherpetic neuralgia.

Topical analgesics for neuropathic pain include lidocaine, which can be administered as a patch and has established efficacy for postherpetic pain (Galer, Rowbotham, Perander, & Friedman, 1999) and anecdotal benefit for other neuropathic pain states (Devers & Galer, 2000); transdermal clonidine (Catapres®), which has an anti-allodynic effect at the site of its application in patients with sympathetically mediated pain (Davis, Treede, Raja, Meyer, & Campbell, 1991); and capsaicin, which needs to be compounded at high concentrations (> 1%) and administered topically under local or regional anesthesia (Robbins et al., 1998). Capsaicin is the natural substance present in hot chili peppers. Recently, a capsaicin-activated neuronal membrane receptor has been cloned (Caterina et al., 1997) and named vanilloid receptor. It is located exclusively on small nerve fibers. After an initial depolarization, the single administration of a large dose of capsaicin appears to produce a prolonged deactivation of the capsaicin-sensitive nociceptors. The analgesic effect is dose-dependent and may last for several weeks. Over-the-counter creams need to be applied several times a day for many weeks. Of note, controlled studies of capsaicin at low concentrations (i.e., 0.075% or less, corresponding to the doses found in over-the-counter preparations) have given mixed results, and this likely is because of the initial burning pain induced by each application. Patient compliance has been poor, and during clinical trials, dropout rates have been high.

Additional Adjuvant Agents
Alpha-2 Adrenergic Agonists

Alpha-2 adrenergic agonists are known to have a spinal antinociceptive effect. Controlled trials have shown the effectiveness of intraspinal clonidine (Catapres®, Duraclon®) for pain control (Eisenach, DuPen, Dubois, Miguel, & Allin, 1995; Khan, Ferguson, & Jones, 1999). Clonidine has been found to potentiate intrathecal opiate analgesia (Pappagallo, 1999). Moreover, transdermal clonidine was found to have a local anti-allodynic effect in patients affected by sympathetically maintained neuropathic pain (Davis et al., 1991).

Tizanidine (Zanaflex®) is a relatively short-acting oral alpha-2 adrenergic agonist with a much lower hypotensive effect than clonidine. Tizanidine has been used for the management of spasticity. However, clinical experience indicates the usefulness of tizanidine for a variety of painful states, including neuropathic pain disorders (Fromm, Aumentado, & Terrence, 1993). The most common side effects of the alpha-2 adrenergic agonists are somnolence and dizziness (to which tolerance usually develops) and clonidine hypotension.

Anti-Inflammatory Drugs and Biphosphonates

Nonsteroidal anti-inflammatory drugs (e.g., cyclo-oxygenase [COX] type 1 and 2 inhibitors, acetaminophen) have been of little benefit in the treatment of neuropathic pain. Steroid therapy may be considered for severe inflammatory pain caused by cancer infiltrating structures like the brachial or lumbosacral plexi, roots, or nerve trunks.

Their analgesic effect may be related to the depletion of activated macrophages and decreased release of pro-inflammatory cytokines in the area of nerve inflammation. In the animal model of neuropathic pain (sciatic nerve ligature), biphosphonates reduced the number of activated macrophages infiltrating the injured nerve, reduced Wallerian nerve fiber degeneration, and decreased experimental hyperalgesia (Liu, Michaelis, Amir, & Devor, 2000).

Gamma-Aminobutyric Acid Agonists

Baclofen (Lioresal®) is an analog of the inhibitory neurotransmitter GABA and has a specific action on the GABA-B receptors. It has been used for many years as an effective spasmolytic agent. Baclofen also has shown effectiveness in the treatment of trigeminal neuralgia (Pappagallo, 1999). Clinical experience supports the use of low-dose baclofen to potentiate the antineuralgic effect of carbamazepine for trigeminal neuralgia. Of note, baclofen also has been used intrathecally to relieve intractable spasticity, and it may have an adjuvant role when added to spinal opiates for the treatment of intractable neuropathic pain and spasticity. The most common side effects of baclofen are drowsiness, weakness, hypotension, and confusion. Discontinuation of baclofen always requires a slow tapering to avoid the occurrence of seizures and other severe neurologic manifestations.

Benzodiazepines (e.g., alprazolam [Xanax®], lorazepam [Ativan®], diazepam [Valium®]) are GABA-A agonists. Their clinical use in patients with chronic pain is controversial (Dellemijn & Fields, 1994; Pappagallo, 1999). In a controlled trial, patients with postherpetic neuralgia did worse on lorazepam than placebo or amitriptyline (Max et al., 1988). Benzodiazepine-related side effects include the onset of depression and disruption of physiologic sleep. In combination with opiates, benzodiazepines cause significant cognitive impairment, whereas opiate analgesics alone do not (Haythornthwaite, Menefee, Quatrano-Piacentini, & Pappagallo, 1998). Moreover, benzodiazepines, when added to an opiate regimen, may favor the development of true tolerance to opiate analgesia (Gear et al., 1997), and clinical experience seems to support this notion.

Invasive Treatment Interventions

Implantable devices, such as intrathecal pumps or spinal cord, motor cortex (Garcia-Larrea et al., 1999), and deep brain stimulators, recently have become available for the treatment of neuropathic pain that responds poorly to standard pharmacologic and conservative therapeutic modalities. Among the most commonly used implantable devices are intrathecal pumps (IPs) and spinal cord stimulators (SCSs). SCSs have been used successfully in patients with intractable limb pain that is not treatable by conventional methods. IPs are used to deliver spinal fluid analgesics such as opiates, clonidine, local anesthetics, and baclofen into the cerebrospinal fluid and will likely be used in the near future for other emerging analgesic agents (e.g., ziconotide, adenosine) (Bennett et al., 2000). Clinical experience and several reports indicate that clonidine or local anesthetics administered intrathecally can potentiate opiate analgesia for neuropathic pain (Katz, 2000). Intrathecal morphine currently is the most commonly used analgesic administered by pump. However, prior to implanting an intrathecal morphine pump, opiate trials need to be performed to show that the patient's pain is somewhat opiate responsive. A pump can be implanted in a permanent fashion after trials are successful. For some specific intractable neuropathic pain disorders, neuroablative procedures might be considered. For example, the dorsal root entry-zone lesion has been recommended for the treatment of intractable pain from brachial plexus avulsions (Thomas & Kitchen, 1994). The decision to perform neuroablative surgery should come only after a thorough comprehensive assessment has been carried out by a multidisciplinary team of pain medicine specialists and conservative management has failed to produce improvement in the patient's quality of life.

Analgesic Stepladder for Neuropathic Pain

The number and variety of options for analgesic treatment of neuropathic pain can be confusing and daunting, even for physicians specializing in the treatment of pain. Polypharmacy and combination treatment employing agents from a variety of pharmacologic classes is the rule, and specific agents can be employed in an escalating regimen that matches the intensity and nature of the neuropathic pain state.

Conclusions

Neuropathic pain states are difficult disorders to treat. Although not yet fully understood, advances are being made in the comprehension of the various mechanisms and etiologies underlying the neuropathic pain syndromes. Patients suffering from these disorders need to have treatment plans tailored to their individual problems. As indicated, a trial of a single medication should be considered initially if the patient presents with mild neuropathic pain and with an overall high level of function. However, as the patient becomes less functional or presents with incapacitating pain, a more aggressive intervention based on a combination of pharmacologic therapies is necessary. Medications—such as ACDs, opiates, antidepressants, and topical agents—along with a rehabilitation medicine program, can help a major portion of patients suffering from these disorders. Implantable devices can aid the patient with intractable disease. Although progress is being made in treating patients with neuropathic pain, it is important to remember that the goals of care always are to (a) perform a comprehensive diagnostic evaluation of the patients; (b) determine the cause of the pain syndrome by obtaining appropriate consultations, if necessary; (c) assess and reassess the clinical and psychosocial status of the patients longitudinally throughout various treatment trials; (d) be supportive without patronizing or telling the patients to "learn how to live with their pain;" and (e) strive for the maximal amount of pain relief that will hopefully allow the patients to have as functional a lifestyle as possible.

References

Baconja, M., Beydoun, A., Edwards, K., Schwartz, S.L., Fonseca, V., Hes, M., LaMoreaux, L., & Garofalo, E. (1998). Gabapentin for the symptomatic treatment of painful neuropathy in patients with diabetes mellitus: A randomized controlled trial. *JAMA, 280,* 1831–1836.

Bennett, G., Deer, T., Du Pen, S., Rauck, R., Yaksh, T., & Hassenbusch, S. (2000). Future directions in the management of pain by intraspinal drug delivery. *Journal of Pain and Symptom Management, 20*(Suppl.), 44–50.

Caterina, M., Schumacher, M., Tominaga, M., Rosen, T.A., Levine, J.D., & Julius, D. (1997). The capsaicin receptor: A heat-activated ion channel in the pain pathway. *Nature, 389,* 816–824.

Davis, K., Treede, R., Raja, S., Meyer, R.A., & Campbell, J.N. (1991). Topical application of clonidine relieves hyperalgesia in patients with sympathetically maintained pain. *Pain, 47,* 309–317.

Dellemijn, P., & Fields, H. (1994). Do benzodiazepines have a role in chronic pain management? *Pain, 57,* 137–152.

Devers, A., & Galer, B. (2000). Topical lidocaine patch relieves a variety of neuropathic pain conditions: An open-label study. *Clinical Journal of Pain, 16,* 205–208.

Eisenach, J., DuPen, S., Dubois, M., Miguel, R., & Allin, D. (1995). Epidural clonidine analgesia for intractable cancer pain. The Epidural Clonidine Study Group. *Pain, 61,* 391–399.

Fromm, G., Aumentado, D., & Terrence, C. (1993). A clinical and experimental investigation of the effects of tizanidine in trigeminal neuralgia. *Pain, 53,* 265–271.

Galer, B., Rowbotham, M., Perander, J., & Friedman, E. (1999). Topical lidocaine patch relieves postherpetic neuralgia more effectively than a vehicle topical patch: Results of an enriched enrollment study. *Pain, 80,* 533–538.

Garcia-Larrea, L., Peyron, R., Mertens, P., Gregoire, M., Lavenne, F., Le Bars, D., Convers, P., Mauguiere, F., Sindou, M., & Laurent, B. (1999). Electrical stimulation of motor cortex for pain control: A combined PET-scan and electrophysiological study. *Pain, 83,* 259–273.

Gear, R., Miaskowski, C., Heller, P., Paul, S., Gordon, N., & Levine, J. (1997). Benzodiazepine mediated antagonism of opioid analgesia. *Pain, 71,* 25–29.

Haythornthwaite, J., Menefee, L., Quatrano-Piacentini, A., & Pappagallo, M. (1998). Outcome of chronic opioid therapy for non-cancer pain. *Journal of Pain and Symptom Management, 15,* 185–194.

Katz, N. (2000). Neuropathic pain in cancer and AIDS. *Clinical Journal of Pain, 16*(Suppl. 2), 41–48.

Khan, Z., Ferguson, C., & Jones, R. (1999). Alpha-2 and imidazoline receptor agonists. Their pharmacology and therapeutic role. *Anaesthesia, 54*(2), 146–165.

Lang, E., Hord, A., & Denson, D. (1996). Venlafaxine hydrochloride (Effexor) relieves thermal hyperalgesia in rats with an experimental mononeuropathy. *Pain, 68,* 151–155.

Liu, C., Michaelis, M., Amir, R., & Devor, M. (2000). Spinal nerve injury enhances subthreshold membrane potential oscillations in DRG neurons: Relation to neuropathic pain. *Journal of Neurophysiology, 84,* 205–215.

Max, M., Lynch, S., Muir, J., Shoaf, S.E., Smoller, B., & Dubner, R. (1992). Effects of desipramine, amitriptyline and fluoxetine on pain in diabetic neuropathy. *New England Journal of Medicine, 326,* 1250–1256.

Max, M., Schafer, S., Culnane, M., Smoller, B., Dubner, R., & Gracely, R. (1988). Amitriptyline, but not lorazepam, relieves postherpetic neuralgia. *Neurology, 38,* 1427–1432.

Pappagallo, M. (1999). Aggressive pharmacologic treatment of pain. *Rheumatic Disease Clinics of North America, 25*(1), 193–213.

Portenoy, R. (1996). Opioid therapy for chronic nonmalignant pain: A review of the critical issues. *Journal of Pain Symptom Management, 11,* 203–217.

Robbins, W., Staats, P., Levine, J., Fields, H.L., Allen, R.W., Campbell, J.N., & Pappagallo, M. (1998). Treatment of intractable pain with topical large doses of capsaicin: Preliminary report. *Anesthesia and Analgesia, 86,* 579–583.

Rowbotham, M., Harden, N., Stacey, B., Bernstein, P., & Magnus-Miller, L. (1998). Gabapentin for the treatment of postherpetic neuralgia: A randomized controlled trial. *JAMA, 280,* 1837–1842.

Schreiber, S., Backer, M., & Pick, C. (1999). The antinociceptive effect of venlafaxine in mice is mediated through opioid and adrenergic mechanisms. *Neuroscience Letters, 273*(2), 85–88.

Suzuki, R., Chapman, V., & Dickenson, A. (1999). The effectiveness of spinal and systemic morphine on rat dorsal horn neuronal responses in the spinal nerve ligation model of neuropathic pain. *Pain, 80,* 215–228.

Thomas, D., & Kitchen, N. (1994). Long-term follow up of dorsal root entry zone lesions in brachial plexus avulsion. *Journal of Neurology, Neurosurgery, and Psychiatry, 57,* 737–738.

Tomlinson, D., Malcangio, M., Patel, J., Meyer, J.B., & Chen, K.S. (1999, October). *Effects of zonisamide on mechanically induced nociception in rats with streptozotocin-diabetes.* Abstract presented at the 18th Annual Scientific Meeting of the American Pain Society, Ft. Lauderdale, FL.

Wallace, M. (2000). Calcium and sodium channel antagonists for the treatment of pain. *Clinical Journal of Pain, 16*(Suppl. 2), 80–85.

Zakrzewska, J., Chaudhry, Z., Nurmikko, T., Patton, D.W., & Mullens, E.L. (1997). Lamotrigine in refractory trigeminal neuralgia: Results from a double-blind placebo controlled crossover trial. *Pain, 73,* 223–230.

Appendix B
Advocacy Competencies
Carol Taylor, CSFN, RN, PhD

Supporting Autonomy

A. Determining and documenting the patient's decision-making capacity, ensuring that agency/institutional policies specify how this is to be performed, and identifying responsible parties

B. Protecting the rights of patients with decision-making capacity to be self-determining
   1. Facilitate communication and documentation of the patient's preferences.
   2. Anticipate the types of treatment decisions that are likely to be needed.
   3. Assist in the preparation of advance directives.

C. Promoting authentic autonomy; authentic decisions reflect the individual's identity, decisional history, and moral norms.

D. Identifying the morally as well as legally valid surrogate decision maker for patients who lack decision-making capacity

E. Supporting the surrogate decision maker and clarifying the surrogate decision maker's role

F. Identifying limits to patient/surrogate autonomy and caregiver autonomy

G. Developing agency/institutional policies that identify the caregivers responsible for and the procedures to be used to identify and support the appropriate decision makers

Promoting Patient Well-Being

A. Clarifying the goal of therapy: Cure and restoration, stabilization of functioning, preparation for a comfortable, dignified death

B. Determining the medical effectiveness of therapy

C. Weighing the benefits and burdens of therapy

D. Ensuring that all interventions are consistent with the overall goal of therapy

E. Ensuring that the patient's priority needs are addressed (biologic, psychosocial, and spiritual needs)

F. Ensuring continuity of care as the patient is transferred among services within and outside of the institution

G. Weighing the moral relevance of third-party (e.g., family, caregiver, institution, society) interests

H. Identifying and addressing forces within society and the healthcare system that compromise patient well-being

Preventing and Resolving Ethical Conflict

A. Establishing that preventing and resolving ethical conflict falls within the authority of all healthcare professionals who are engaged in the care of a patient

B. Developing awareness of and sensitivity to the conscious and unconscious sources of conflict

C. Facilitating timely communication among those involved in decision making: one-on-one meetings and periodic meetings of the patient, family, and interdisciplinary team to clarify goals and plan of care

D. Documenting pertinent information on the patient record

E. Referring unresolved ethical issues to the ethics consult team or the institutional ethics committee

F. Identifying and addressing system variables that are contributing to recurrent ethical problems

Appendix C
Internet Resources

Sources for Specific Assessment Tools

www.palliative.org—includes the Edmonton Symptom Assessment Scale, numeric assessment of various symptoms, the CAGE Questionnaire to determine a positive substance use history, the Home Care Assessment Tool, and Mini Mental Examination

www.cher.brown.edu/pcoc/toolkit.htm—includes a "tool kit" containing various instruments and outcome measurements for quality of care at the end of life.

Sources Specific to Pain Management

www.ahcpr.gov/clinic/index.html—U.S. Public Health Service, Agency for Healthcare Research and Quality, includes access to federal guidelines for the management of acute pain and cancer pain

www.ampainsoc.org—American Pain Society and the American Academy of Pain Medicine. Consensus statement on the use of opiates in chronic pain.

www.americangeriatrics.org/products/chronic_pain.pdf—American Geriatrics Society's Clinical Practice Guideline, *The Management of Chronic Pain in Older Persons*

www.asam.org—The American Society of Addiction Medicine's public policy statement

www.iasp-pain.org—International Association for the Study of Pain

www.pain.com—World Congress on Pain

www.bmj.com/cgi/collection/pain—*British Medical Journal*'s articles on pain

General End-of-Life Care Resources

www.abcd-caring.org—Americans for Better Care of the Dying

www.medicaring.org—Center to Improve the Care of the Dying

www.growthhouse.org—Growth House, Inc.

www.edc.org/lastacts—Innovations in End-of-Life Care

www.promotingexcellence.org—Promoting Excellence in End-of-Life Care

www.careofdying.org—Supportive Care of the Dying

www.ama-assn.org/ethic—American Medical Association Curriculum for End-of-Life Care

www.lastacts.org—Last Acts: A Coalition to Improve Care and Caring Near the End of Life

www.nhpco.org—National Hospice and Palliative Care Organization

www.partnershipforcaring.org—Partnership for Caring: America's Voices For the Dying

www.soros.org/death.html—Open Society Institute Project on Death in America

www.epec.net—Education for Physicians on End of Life Care

www.capcmssm.org—Center to Advance Palliative Care

www.dyingwell.com—Dying Well

Resources Specific to Nursing

www.hpna.org—Hospice and Palliative Nurses Association

www.ons.org—Oncology Nursing Society

Pharmaceutical Agents Used in This Text

Provided below are the generic names, trade names, and manufacturers of pharmaceutical agents appearing in this text.

Pharmaceutical Agents Used in This Text

Generic Name	Trade Name	Manufacturer
Acetaminophen	Tylenol	McNeil Consumer, Fort Washington, PA
Acetylsalicylic acid	Aspirin	Bayer Consumer Care, Parsipanny, NJ
Acyclovir	Zovirax	GlaxoSmithKline, Research Triangle Park, NC
Albuterol	Proventil	Schering, Kenilworth, NJ
Alprazolam	Xanax	Pharmacia & Upjohn, Kalamazoo, MI
Amitriptyline	Elavil	AstraZeneca, Wilmington, DE
Ampicillin	Amoxil	GlaxoSmithKline, Research Triangle Park, NC
Azithromycin	Zithromax	Pfizer, New York, NY
Baclofen	Lioresal	Rosemont Pharmaceuticals, Denver, CO
Beclomethasone	Beclovent	GlaxoSmithKline, Research Triangle Park, NC
Benzonatate	Tessalon Perles	Forest Pharmaceuticals, St. Louis, MO
Bisacodyl	Dulcolax	GlaxoSmithKline, Research Triangle Park, NC
Bethanechol	Urecholine	Merck, West Point, PA
Bupivicaine	Marcaine	AstraZeneca, Wilmington, DE
Buspirone	BuSpar	Bristol-Myers Squibb, Princeton, NJ
Capsaicin	Zostrix	GenDerm, Lincolnshire, IL
Carbamazepine	Tegretol	Novartis, East Hanover, NJ

(Continued on next page)

Pharmaceutical Agents Used in This Text (Continued)

Generic Name	Trade Name	Manufacturer
Casanthrol and docusate sodium	Peri-Colace	Roberts Pharmaceuticals, Eatontown, NJ
Cephalexin	Keflex	Dista Products, Indianapolis, IN
Chlorazepate	Tranxene	Abbott, Abbott Park, IL
Chlorothiazide	Diuril	Merck, West Point, PA
Chlorpromazine	Thorazine	GlaxoSmithKline, Research Triangle Park, NC
Cholestyramine	Questran	Upsher-Smith, Minneapolis, MN
Cimetidine	Tagamet	GlaxoSmithKline, Research Triangle Park, NC
Ciprofloxacin	Cipro	Bayer Pharmaceuticals, Westhaven, CT
Clonazepam	Klonopin	Roche, Nutley, NJ
Clonidine	Catapres Duraclon	Boehringer Ingelheim, Ridgefield, CT
Codeine	Multiple brands	Multiple manufacturers
Collagenase	Santyl	Knoll, Whippany, NJ
Cylert	Pemoline	Abbott, Abbott Park, IL
Cyproheptadine hydro-chloride	Periactin	Merck, West Point, PA
Demeclocycline	Declomycin	Lederle, Philadelphia, PA
Desipramine	Norpramin	Aventis Pharmaceuticals, Kansas City, MO
Dexamethasone	Decadron	Merck, West Point, PA
Dextroamphetamine	Dexedrine	GlaxoSmithKline, Research Triangle Park, NC
Diazepam	Valium	Roche, Nutley, NJ
Diphenhydramine	Benadryl	Warner-Lambert, Morris Plains, NJ
Docusate sodium	Colace	Roberts Pharmaceuticals, Eatontown, NJ
Dronabinol	Marinol	Roxane, Columbus, OH
Droperidol	Inapsine	Johnson & Johnson, New Brunswick, NJ
Erythromycin	E-Mycin	Knoll, Whippany, NJ
Famciclovir	Famvir	GlaxoSmithKline, Research Triangle Park, NC
Fentanyl	Duragesic	Janssen Pharmaceuticals, Titusville, NJ
Fibrinolysin	Elase	Fujisawa, Deerfield, IL
Fluconazole	Diflucan	Pfizer Laboratories, New York, NY

(Continued on next page)

Pharmaceutical Agents Used in This Text *(Continued)*

Generic Name	Trade Name	Manufacturer
Fluoxetine	Prozac	Eli Lilly, Indianapolis, IN
Furosemide	Lasix	Aventis Pharmaceuticals, Kansas City, MO
Gabapentin	Neurontin	Parke Davis, Morris Plains, NJ
Glycopyrrolate	Robinul	First Horizon Pharmaceuticals, Roswell, GA
Haloperidol	Haldol	Ortho-McNeil Pharmaceuticals, Raritan, NJ
Hyaluronidase	Wydase	Wyeth-Ayerst, Philadelphia, PA
Hydrocodone	Vicodin	Knoll, Whippany, NJ
Hydromorphone	Dilaudid	Knoll, Whippany, NJ
Hydroxyzine hydrochloride	Atarax	Pfizer, New York, NY
Hyoscyamine sulfate	Levsin	Schwarz Pharma, Mequon, WI
Ibuprofen	Motrin	Pharmacia & Upjohn, Kalamazoo, MI
Imipramine	Tofranil	Novartis, East Hanover, NJ
Ipratropium	Atrovent	Boehringer Ingelheim, Ridgefield, CT
Isoproterenol	Isuprel	Sterling Drug, Wilmington, DE
Lactulose	Chronulac	Aventis Pharmaceuticals, Kansas City, MO
Lamotrigine	Lamictal	GlaxoSmithKline, Research Triangle Park, NC
Levetiracetam	Keppra	UCB Pharma, Smyrna, GA
Lorazepam	Ativan	Wyeth-Ayerst, Philadelphia, PA
Megestrol	Megace	Mead Johnson, Princeton, NJ
Metaproterenol	Alupent	Boehringer Ingelheim, Ridgefield, CT
Methadone	Dolophine	Eli Lilly, Indianapolis, IN
Methylphenidate	Ritalin	Novartis, East Hanover, NJ
Methylprednisolone	Medrol	Pharmacia & Upjohn, Kalamazoo, MI
Metoclopramide	Reglan	Whitehall-Robins Healthcare, Madison, NJ
Metronidazole	Flagyl	Searle, Skokie, IL
Mexiletine	Mexitil	Boehringer Ingelheim, Ridgefield, CT
Midazolam	Versed	Roche, Nutley, NJ
Mirtazapine	Remeron	Organon, West Orange, NJ
Morphine sulfate	Multiple brands	Multiple manufacturers based on preparation

(Continued on next page)

Pharmaceutical Agents Used in This Text *(Continued)*

Generic Name	Trade Name	Manufacturer
Neostigmine methysulfate	Prostigmin	Roche, Nutley, NJ
Nifedipine	Procardia	Pratt Pharmaceuticals, New York, NY
Nitrofurantoin	Macrodantin	Proctor & Gamble, Cincinnati, OH
Nortriptyline	Aventyl Pamelor	Eli Lilly, Indianapolis, IN Novartis, East Hanover, NJ
Nystatin	Mycostatin	Bristol-Myers Squibb, Princeton, NJ
Octreotide	Sandostatin	Novartis, East Hanover, NJ
Olanzapine	Zyprexa	Eli Lilly, Indianapolis, IN
Ondansetron	Zofran	GlaxoSmithKline, Research Triangle Park, NC
Oxcarbazepine	Trileptal	Novartis, East Hanover, NJ
Oxybutynin	Ditropan	Alza, Palo Alto, CA
Oxycodone	Roxicodone	Roxane, Columbus, OH
Oxycodone-acetaminophen	Percocet	Endo Pharmaceuticals, Chadds Ford, PA
Pamidronate	Aredia	Novartis, East Hanover, NJ
Pancrelipase	Viokase	Axcan Scandipharm, Birmingham, AL
Papain urea	Accuzyme	Healthpoint, Fort Worth, TX
Paroxetine	Paxil	GlaxoSmithKline, Research Triangle Park, NC
Phenazopyridine	Pyridium	Parke Davis, Morris Plains, NJ
Phenobarbital	Donnatal	A.H. Robins, Richmond, VA
Phenytoin	Dilantin	Parke Davis, Morris Plains, NJ
Pilocarpine	Salagen	MGI Pharma, Bloomington, MN
Prednisone	Deltasone	Pharmacia & Upjohn, Kalamazoo, MI
Prochlorperazine	Compazine	GlaxoSmithKline, Research Triangle Park, NC
Promethazine	Phenergan	Wyeth-Ayerst Laboratories, Philadelphia, PA
Quetiapine	Seroquel	AstraZeneca, Wilmington, DE
Risperidone	Risperdal	Janssen Pharmaceutica, Titusville, NJ
Saline enema	Fleet [enema]	C.B. Fleet, Lynchburg, VA
Scopolamine	Transderm-Scop	Novartis, East Hanover, NJ
Senna	Senokot	Purdue Frederick, Norwalk, CT
Sertraline	Zoloft	Pfizer Laboratories, New York, NY

(Continued on next page)

Pharmaceutical Agents Used in This Text *(Continued)*

Generic Name	Trade Name	Manufacturer
Sildenafil	Viagra	Pfizer Laboratories, New York, NY
Simethicone	Maalox Plus	Aventis Pharmaceuticals, Kansas City, MO
Spironolactone	Aldactone	Searle, Skokie, IL
Temazepam	Restoril	Novartis, East Hanover, NJ
Theophylline	Theo-Dur	Schering, Kenilworth, NJ
Tiagabine	Gabitril	Cephalon, West Chester, PA
Tizanidine	Zanaflex	Elan Pharmaceuticals, Dublin, Ireland
Tramadol	Ultram	Ortho-McNeil Pharmaceuticals, Raritan, NJ
Triazolam	Halcion	Pharmacia & Upjohn, Kalamazoo, MI
Trimethobenzamide	Tigan	Roche, Nutley, NJ
Trimethoprim-sulfamethoxazole	Bactrim Cotrim	Roberts Pharmaceutical, Eatontown, NJ GlaxoSmithKline, Research Triangle Park, NC
Valacyclovir	Valtrex	GlaxoSmithKline, Research Triangle Park, NC
Valproic acid	Depakene	Abbott, North Chicago, IL
Venlafaxine	Effexor	Wyeth-Ayerst Pharmaceuticals, St. Davids, PA
Xylocaine	Lidocaine	AstraZeneca, Wilmington, DE
Zolendronate	Zometa	Novartis, East Hanover, NJ
Zolpidem	Ambien	Searle, Skokie, IL
Zonisamide	Zonegran	Elan Pharmaceuticals, Dublin, Ireland

Note. This list is not comprehensive; more than one company may manufacture or market a product known by the same generic name. Although every effort was made to ensure the accuracy of this information at press time, product marketing changes frequently, as do brand names; therefore, the publisher and contributors disclaim responsibility for the accuracy of this list.

Glossary

Acupuncture. An Asian practice that uses the insertion of fine needles into innervated body areas to illicit analgesia.

Addiction. Both physical and psychologic cravings that result in the continued use of specific substances or drugs (prescribed or illicit) despite harm.

Adjuvant analgesic drug. Medications that have primary purposes other than pain management, but when they are combined with an opiate analgesic, they produce optimal analgesia.

Advance directive. Identification of an individual's healthcare goals and guidance regarding his or her future treatment options.

Advanced illness. A chronic malignant or nonmalignant disease that no longer responds to curative biomedical interventions. Advanced illness is considered the point along the disease trajectory when care should focus on palliative versus curative interventions.

Adverse effects. Individual variations, in the response to endogenous medications, that interfere with quality of life.

Advocate. A person selected by the patient to implement advance directives in the event that the patient is unable to advocate for himself or herself. The role of the advocate is conferred through durable power of attorney.

Allodynia. The result of extreme dermal neuropathic pain—the patient is unable to tolerate touch or pressure on or sensation in the affected skin area.

Automation of Reports and Consolidated Orders System. An automated, comprehensive drug-reporting system that monitors controlled substances from the point of manufacture through sales and distribution. This monitoring occurs through the U.S. Department of Justice Drug Enforcement Administration.

Best-evidence synthesis. Information based upon the best-evidence principle frequently used in law. Best-evidence synthesis suggests that the evidence that would be essential in one case may be disregarded in a second case in the event that better evidence becomes available.

Cardiopulmonary resuscitation (CPR). A physical skill that involves giving artificial respiration and chest compressions to a person whose breathing and heart have stopped.

Caregiver. Someone who is responsible for attending to the functional needs of an ill person. An informal caregiver is not paid, usually a member of the family or a friend; a formal caregiver is paid and has undergone specific education and training.

Chilling effect. The influence on healthcare providers' actions that are a result of perceived (real or unreal) regulatory or disciplinary actions affecting their prescribing practices.

Chronic pain. Pain that does not have a predictable course, usually extends beyond six months, and is caused by various etiologies both malignant and nonmalignant.

Controlled Substances Act. A federal law, formally called Title II of the Comprehensive Drug Abuse Prevention and Control Act of 1970 (21 United States Code). This law consolidated numerous laws regulating the manufacture and distribution of opiates, psychostimulants, antidepressants, hallucinogens, anabolic steroids, and pharmaceuticals used in the production of controlled substances. For more information, visit the U.S. Department of Justice, Drug Enforcement Administration Web site at www.usdoj.gov/dea/concern/abuse/chap1/contents.htm.

Counterstimulant. The use of sensory stimulation—such as cold, heat, rubbing, pressure, or electrical current—to help decrease the pain perception. Can be used alone or with an opiate.

Curative care. Traditional biomedical approach to the treatment of disease—active and aggressive interventions with the goal of curing the patient.

Disciplinary action. Censure by a professional licensing board, as the result of an individual licensee's violation of statute or rules.

Diversion. Using medications for recreational, financial, or illegal purposes.

Do not resuscitate order. A physician's or individual's explicitly written instructions not to attempt cardiopulmonary resuscitation in case of cardiac or respiratory arrest.

Doctor shopper. A person who is perceived as going from physician to physician to obtain medications.

Drug. A chemical compound used or ingested to solicit desired outcomes.

Drug Abuse Warning Network. A federal program that uses medical records to monitor national drug abuse trends and adverse health effects from various medications.

Drug Enforcement Administration, U.S. Department of Justice. The federal agency that is responsible for the enforcement of controlled substance laws and regulations.

End-of-life care. The "umbrella term" that covers both palliative and hospice care. In the United States, this is influenced by reimbursement issues.

Equianalgesic. Describes how one medication or the route of adminstration is equally effective to another.

Eutectic mixture of local anesthetic. An ointment matrix that contains local anesthetics and is applied topically.

Family. Identified by the patient and can include familial relatives, spouse, life partners, unrelated friends, and informal caregivers.

Healing. To restore health, mend, or impart a sense of well-being. Includes the many dimensions of the patient.

Hospice care. Uses an interdisciplinary approach of care based upon the patient's and family's goals. The patient must have a life-limited prognosis of six months or fewer. Hospice views death as a normal experience.

Hyperalgesia. Occurs when opiate therapy becomes toxic as a result of too much medication or because of symptoms, such as renal failure or dehydration.

Illegal drug/narcotic. Medications (e.g., heroin) that have therapeutic benefits but are used instead for recreational purposes.

Loading dose. An aggressive dosage of a specific medication to promote active bioavailability of the medication to improve a patient's symptoms.

Maintenance dose. Patient-specific dosage that has been titrated to control pain and symptoms.

Mixed opiate agonist-antagonist. A compound that has an affinity for two or more types of opioid receptors and blocks opiate effects on one receptor type while producing opiate effects on a second receptor type.

Narcotic. A narcotic is an illegal drug. The term *narcotic* is no longer used in medical literature, which now uses *opiate*.

Nonsteroidal anti-inflammatory drug (NSAID). Drug that reduces inflammation (and hence pain) arising from injured tissue.

- Nonselective NSAID: An NSAID that inhibits both COX1 and COX2 isoforms of cyclo-oxygenase.

- COX 2-selective NSAID: An NSAID that inhibits the COX2 isoform of cyclo-oxygenase but not the C1 form.

Opiate. Opiates are found in all analgesics—both Class II and III. Opiates bind to the mu receptor sites within the central nervous system and block the pain perception between the periphery and the brain (the gate effect). Opiates are both therapeutic and essential to control pain.

Opiate receptors. Opiate-binding sites found throughout the central nervous system and the gastrointestinal tract.

Pain. A multidimensional, unpleasant sensory experience associated with actual or potential tissue damage.

Pain, acute. Pain with a predictable course and treatment—a relatively straightforward, temporary affliction.

Pain affect. The emotional dimension of the pain experience.

Pain, neuropathic. Results from a disturbance of function or pathologic change in a nerve; in one nerve, mononeuropathy; in several nerves, mononeuropathy multiplex; if diffuse and bilateral, polyneuropathy. Most frequently associated with other pain syndromes, such as somatic and visceral.

Palliative care. Provides expertise in pain and symptom management, versus curative care, for patients living and dying with advanced illness. It is interdisciplinary and begins early in the course of illness. Palliative care is a medical specialty in many countries and is newly developing in the United States.

Peer review. Critical evaluation, by experts in the author's field, of an author's work. Ensures competent research-based publications or resources.

Physical dependence. The condition that exists if, when a specific medication is suddenly withdrawn, the patient experiences adverse effects.

Physical modalities. Exogenous and nonpharmaceutic interventions—such as heat, cold, massage, aromatherapy, color, and music—used in combination with therapeutic medications.

Pseudoaddiction. Drug-seeking behavior that occurs because a patient's pain is not adequately managed.

Regulatory complaint. A mechanism for consumers to file, with a state licensing agency, their criticisms or objections to procedures or care provided by licensed healthcare providers (e.g., physicians, nurses, dentists, pharmacists, licensed healthcare institutions or systems [nursing homes, home health agencies, hospices, hospitals, freestanding surgical units, ambulatory surgical units, end-stage renal dialysis centers]). The agency receives and processes such complaints by following specific guidelines and processes established by statutes or rules.

Respite care. Temporary care provided so a patient's caregiver can have personal time outside of the demands of the patient's care.

Schedule I drugs. This group includes heroin, LSD, and marijuana. Schedule I drugs have the following characteristics: (a) the drug or other substance has a high potential for abuse; (b) the drug or other substance has no currently accepted medical use in treatment in the United States; and (c) there is a lack of accepted safety for the use of the drug or other substance under medical supervision (Controlled Substances Act of 1970: see www.mpp .org/statelaw/app_e.html).

Schedule II drugs. This group includes dronabinol, methadone, morphine, methamphetamine, and cocaine. Schedule II drugs have the following characteristics: (a) the drug or other substance has a high potential for abuse; (b) the drug or other substance has a currently accepted medical use in treatment in the United States or a currently accepted medical use with severe restrictions; (c) abuse of the drug or other substance may lead to severe psychologic or physical dependence (Controlled Substances Act of 1970: see www.mpp.org/ statelaw/app_e.html).

Schedule III drugs. This group includes anabolic steroids. Schedule III drugs have the following characteristics: (a) the drug or other substance has a potential of abuse less than the drugs or other substances in Schedules I and II; (b) the drug or other substance has a currently accepted medical use in treatment in the United States; (c) abuse of the drug or other substance may lead to moderate or low physical dependence or high psychologic dependence (Controlled Substances Act of 1970: see www.mpp.org/statelaw/app_e.html).

Schedule IV drugs. This group includes diazepam and other tranquilizers. Schedule IV drugs have the following characteristics: (a) the drug or other substance has a low potential for abuse relative to the drugs or other substances in Schedule III; (b) the drug or other substance has a currently accepted medical use in treatment in the United States; (c) abuse of the drug or other substance may lead to limited physical dependence or psychologic dependence relative to the drugs or other substances in Schedule III (Controlled Substances Act of 1970: see www.mpp.org/statelaw/app_e.html).

Schedule V drugs. This group includes codeine-containing analgesics. Schedule V drugs have the following characteristics: (a) the drug or other substance has a low potential for abuse relative to the drugs or other substances in Schedule IV; (b) the drug or other substance has a currently accepted medical use in treatment in the United States; (c) abuse of the drug or other substance may lead to limited physical dependence or psychologic dependence relative to the drugs or other substances in Schedule IV (Controlled Substances Act of 1970: see www.mpp.org/statelaw/app_e.html).

Suffering. A state of severe distress associated with events that threaten the intactness of the person.

Terminal illness. Defined by the Medicare hospice benefit as an illness from which the patient has fewer than six months of a life-limited diagnosis.

Terminal sedation. Sedation that uses high doses of pharmaceutical, to provide comfort for unrelenting symptoms.

Titrate. To gradually increase or decrease medication to produce optimal outcomes—very patient specific. Titrating also is called tapering.

Transcutaneous electrical nerve stimulation. A method of producing electroanalgesia through electrodes applied to the skin.

Tolerance. A state of physiologic adaptation after prolonged exposure to a specific drug or substance.

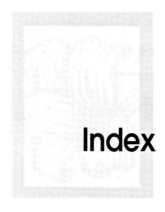

Index

The letter *t* after a page number indicates a table; the letter *f* indicates a figure.

A

Abandonment, fear of, 165, 205
Abdominal pain, with bowel obstruction, 39
Accuzyme. *See* Papain urea
ACDs. *See* Anticonvulsant drugs
Acetaminophen (Tylenol)
    for fever, 124
    for pain, 187
Acetic acid solution, for pressure ulcers,
    223
Acetylsalicylic acid, for fever, 124
Acupuncture, 55
    definition of, 265
    for xerostomia, 244
Acute pain, definition of, 268
Acyclovir (Zovirax), for zoster, 245
Addict, definition of, 170
Addiction, definition of, 265
Adjustment disorder, reactive anxiety, 23
Adjuvant analgesic agents, 189–190, 189*t*
    definition of, 265
    for neuropathic pain, 249–250
Advanced illness, definition of, 265
Advance directives, 1–4
    communication about, 48
    definition of, 1, 265
    family and, 112
    implementation of, 2–3
    and nutrition decisions, 19
    and travel, 235–236

Adverse effects, definition of, 265
Advocate, definition of, 265
After-Death Bereavement Family Interview,
    197
Aging of population, and palliative care,
    193
Aging With Dignity, 4
Agitation, 5–7
    definition of, 5
    management of, 6, 9–10
    manifestations of, 5–6, 9
    pathophysiology/etiology of, 5
Albumin, with paracentesis, 28
Albuterol (Proventil), for dyspnea, 98
Aldactone. *See* Spironolactone
Allodynia, definition of, 265
Alpha-2 adrenergic agonists, for neuro-
    pathic pain, 249
Alprazolam (Xanax)
    for anxiety, 24
    for neuropathic pain, 250
Alupent. *See* Metaproterenol
AMA. *See* American Medical Association
Ambien. *See* Zolpidem
American Association of Health Plans, 163
American Medical Association (AMA)
    Code of Ethics, 19
    Council on Ethical and Judicial Affairs,
        on advance directives, 2
American Nurses Association (ANA), on
        advance directives, 2

Amitriptyline (Elavil)
   for depression, 86*t*
   for neuropathic pain, 248
   in pain management, 189*t*
Ampicillin (Amoxil), for infection, 152
ANA. *See* American Nurses Association
Analgesic stepladder for neuropathic pain,
      251
Analgesics, 188*t*
   for bowel obstruction, 40
   for neuropathic pain, 248–249
   and sexual problems, 217
Anemia, 9–11
   definition of, 9
   pathophysiology/etiology of, 9
Anointing, 53
Anorexia, 13–22
   definition of, 13
   management of, 14–17
   pathophysiology/etiology of, 13
Antacids, and constipation, 59
Antibiotics
   for fever, 124
   for infection, 152–153
   and nausea, 179
Anticholinergics
   for bowel obstruction, 40
   and constipation, 59
   during dying process, 74
   for dyspnea, 98
   for nausea and vomiting, 181*t*
Anticipatory grief, 130
Anticonvulsant drugs (ACDs)
   and constipation, 59
   for hiccups, 134
   and nausea, 179
   for neuropathic pain, 247
   in pain management, 189, 189*t*
Antidepressants, 86–87. *See also* Tricyclic
      antidepressants
   classifications of, 86*t*
   and delirium, 81
   for insomnia, 156
   in pain management, 189–190, 189*t*
Antidiarrheal medications, 90
Antidiuretic hormone, inappropriate
      secretion of (SIADH), 101
   manifestations of, 101
Antiemetics, 181*t*
   for bowel obstruction, 40

Antiepileptics. *See* Anticonvulsant drugs
Antihistamines, for pruritus, 200
Antihypertensive agents, and constipation,
      59
Antipsychotics, for anxiety, 25
Antipyretics, 124
Antiulcer medications, 94
Anxiety, 23–26
   definition of, 23
   versus fear, 119
   management of, 24–25
   manifestations of, 24
   pathophysiology/etiology of, 23–24
   versus spiritual need, 227
Anxiolytics
   for anxiety, 25
   and delirium, 82
   for dyspnea, 98
   for insomnia, 156
Appetite, poor, management of, 14–15
Aredia. *See* Pamidronate
Aromatherapy, 52–53
Art therapy, 55
Ascites, 27–30
   definition of, 27
   management of, 28–29
   manifestations of, 27–28
   pathophysiology/etiology of, 27
Aspirin, for fever, 124
Asthenia, 31–33
   definition of, 31
   management of, 32
   manifestations of, 31
   pathophysiology/etiology of, 31
Atarax. *See* Hydroxyzine hydrochloride
Ativan. *See* Lorazepam
Atomizer, for aromatherapy, 53
Atropine
   during dying process, 74
   for dyspnea, 98
Atrovent. *See* Ipratropium
Automation of Reports and Consolidated
      Orders System, definition of,
      265
Autonomy
   and ethics, 106*t*
   and quality of life, 208
   supporting, 255
Azithromycin (Zithromax), for infection,
      152

B

Baclofen (Lioresal)
  for hiccups, 134
  for neuropathic pain, 250
Bactrim. *See* Trimethoprim/
  sulfamethoxazole
Barbiturates, for seizures, 212
Baths, hydrotherapy, 52
Beclomethasone (Beclovent), for dyspnea,
  98
Benadryl. *See* Diphenhydramine
Beneficence, and ethics, 106*t*
Benzodiazepines
  and agitation, 6
  for anxiety, 24
  and delirium, 82
  for dyspnea, 98
  for nausea and vomiting, 181*t*
  for neuropathic pain, 250
  for seizures, 212
Benzonatate (Tessalon Perles), for cough, 64
Bereavement, 35–37
  definition of, 35
Bergamot *(Citrus bergamia)* oil, 52*t*
Best-evidence synthesis, definition of, 265
Bethanechol (Urecholine), for dysphagia,
  94
Bisacodyl (Dulcolax), for constipation, 61
Bisphosphonates
  for hypercalcemia, 180
  for pain, 190
  in pain management, 189*t*
Bleeding, of skin lesions, controlling, 224
Bloating, management of, 14
Blood (product) transfusions
  for anemia, 10
  for asthenia, 32
  for dyspnea, 98
  for fatigue, 116
Bowel obstruction, 39
  definition of, 39
  management of, 40
  manifestations of, 39–40
  pathophysiology/etiology of, 39
BRAT diet, 90
Breakthrough pain
  definition of, 185
  management of, 188
Bronchodilators, for dyspnea, 98

Bupivicaine (Marcaine), for cough, 64
Buspirone (BuSpar), for anxiety, 25
Butyrophenones, for nausea and vomiting,
  181*t*

C

Cachexia, 13–22
  definition of, 13
  management of, 14–17
  manifestations of, 13–14
  pathophysiology/etiology of, 13
Calcitonin, for hypercalcemia, 180
Cancer
  cachexia in, 13
  small lung cell, and edema, 101
Candles, for aromatherapy, 53
Cannabinoids
  for anorexia, 18
  for nausea and vomiting, 181*t*
  in pain management, 189*t,* 190
Capsaicin (Zostrix)
  for neuropathic pain, 249
  for zoster, 246
Carbamazepine (Tegretol)
  for hiccups, 134
  for neuropathic pain, 247
  in pain management, 189*t*
  for seizures, 212
Cardiopulmonary resuscitation (CPR),
  definition of, 266
Care-based approach, to ethics, 106–107
Caregiver(s)
  and abandonment, 166
  and cultural awareness, 68
  definition of, 43, 266
  education on quality of life, 208
  hopelessness in, 144–145
  and legal issues in pain management,
    169–173
  outcomes for, 45
Caregiver burden, 43–45
  definition of, 43
  funeral planning and, 127
Casanthrol and docusate sodium
    (Peri-Colace), for constipation, 60
Catapres. *See* Clonidine
Catheter
  Foley, 240
  Tenckhoff, 29

Catheter infections, treatment of, 153
Catheters
    for ascites, 29
    during dying process, 73
Cephalexin (Keflex), for lymphedema, 176
Chalice of response, 55
Chemotherapy
    and anemia, 9
    for dyspnea, 98
    for malignant cutaneous wounds, 223
    and massage, 52
Chilling effect, definition of, 266
Chlorazepate (Tranxene), for anxiety, 24
Chlorpromazine (Thorazine)
    for anxiety, 25
    for delirium, 82
    for hiccups, 134
    for nausea and vomiting, 181*t,* 182
    for terminal sedation, 233
Chlorthiazide (Diuril), for dyspnea, 98
Choice in Dying, 4
Cholestyramine (Questran), for pruritus,
    200
Chronic pain, definition of, 266
Chronulac. *See* Lactulose
Cimetidine (Tagamet), for pruritus, 200
Ciprofloxacin (Cipro), for infection, 152
Citrus bergamia (bergamot), 52*t*
Civil proceedings, on pain management,
    172–173
Clonazepam (Klonopin)
    for anxiety, 24
    for terminal sedation, 233
Clonidine (Catapres; Duraclon), for
    neuropathic pain, 249
Codeine, 188*t*
    for cough, 64
Codes of ethics, 107
Cognitive function, maintaining, versus
    symptom control, 207
Colace. *See* Docusate sodium
Collagenase (Santyl), for skin lesions, 223
Comfort
    in dying process, 72
    for fever, 124
    for travel, 236
Common good approach, to ethics, 106
Communication, 47–50
    about funeral planning, 127–128
    about sexuality, 216

about spirituality, 229
    barriers to, 47–48
    cultural dissonance and, 67
    ethics and, 105
    family and, 111
    and psychologic support, 204
    strategies for, 48–49
Community resources
    for caregiver support, 44–45
    for coverage, 162–163
Compazine. *See* Prochlorperazine
Complementary therapies (CTs), 51–57
    definition of, 51
    evaluating appropriateness of, 51–52
    methods of, 52–55
Complex decongestive physiotherapy, for
    lymphedema, 176
Complicated grief, 130
Compress, for aromatherapy, 53
Compression garments
    for edema, 102
    for lymphedema, 176
Compression pumps, for lymphedema, 176
Confusion, acute, 81–83
    management of, 82
    manifestations of, 81–82
    pathophysiology/etiology of, 81
Conscious sedation, definition of, 266
Constipation, 59–61
    definition of, 59
    management of, 60–61
    manifestations of, 59–60
    pain management and, 190
    pathophysiology/etiology of, 59
Continuous care, in hospice, 148
Control, and quality of life, 208
Controlled Substances Act (CSA), 170
    definition of, 266
Coping skills, 203
    and bereavement, 35
    family and, 113
    spiritual, 228
Corticosteroids
    for anorexia, 18
    for bowel obstruction, 40
    for dyspnea, 98
    for nausea and vomiting, 181*t*
    in pain management, 189*t,* 190
Co-trimoxazole (Cotrim), for *Pneumocystis
    carinii* infection, 152

Cough, 63–65
    definition of, 63
    management of, 63–64
    manifestations of, 63
    pathophysiology/etiology of, 63
Counseling
    for fear, 120
    on sexuality, 217–218
Counterstimulant, definition of, 266
CPR. *See* Cardiopulmonary resuscitation
Crescendo pain, 81
CSA. *See* Controlled Substances Act
CTs. *See* Complementary therapies
Cultural awareness, 67–69
    definition of, 67
    strategies for, 68
Cultural dissonance, 67
Culture
    and communication, 48–49
    and family issues, 112
    and hope, 144
Cupressus sempervirens (cypress), 52*t*
Curative care, definition of, 266
Cylert (Pemoline), for asthenia, 32
Cypress *(Cupressus sempervirens)* oil, 52*t*
Cyproheptadine hydrochloride (Periactin),
    for anorexia, 18
Cytokines, and cachexia, 13

D

Dakin's solution, for pressure ulcers, 223
DEA. *See* Drug Enforcement Administra-
    tion
Death, 71–75
    definition of, 71
    quality of life and, 207
Debridement, for pressure ulcers, 223–224
Decadron. *See* Dexamethasone
Decision making, family and, 113
Declomycin. *See* Demeclocycline
Dehydration, 77–79
    definition of, 77
    in dying process, 19
    management of, 78
    manifestations of, 77–78
    pathophysiology/etiology of, 77
Delirium, 81–83
    definition of, 81
    management of, 82

    manifestations of, 81–82
    and nausea, 182
    pathophysiology/etiology of, 81
Deltasone. *See* Prednisone
Demeclocycline (Declomycin), for edema,
    102
Dementia, definition of, 81
Denial, and communication, 47–48
Denver ascites shunts, for ascites, 29
Depakene. *See* Valproic acid
Depression, 85–88
    definition of, 85
    management of, 86–87
    manifestations of, 85–86
    pathophysiology/etiology of, 85
Desipramine (Norpramin)
    for neuropathic pain, 248
    in pain management, 189*t*
Dexamethasone (Decadron)
    for bowel obstruction, 40
    for dyspnea, 98
    for nausea and vomiting, 181*t,* 182
    in pain management, 189*t,* 190
Dextroamphetamine (Dexedrine)
    for asthenia, 32
    for depression, 86, 86*t,* 87
Diarrhea, 89–91
    definition of, 89
    enteral feeding and, 17*t*
    management of, 89–90
    manifestations of, 89
    pathophysiology/etiology of, 89
Diazepam (Valium)
    for anxiety, 24
    for neuropathic pain, 250
    for seizures, 212
    for terminal sedation, 233
Dietary guidelines, for diarrhea, 90
Diffuser, for aromatherapy, 53
Diflucan. *See* Fluconazole
Digoxin
    and delirium, 81
    and nausea, 179
Dilantin. *See* Phenytoin
Dilaudid. *See* Hydromorphone
Diphenhydramine (Benadryl)
    for nausea and vomiting, 182
    for pruritus, 200
    for terminal sedation, 233
Disciplinary action, definition of, 266

Discomfort, versus spiritual need, 227
Disease progression, and quality of life, 208
Distress thermometer, 87
Diuretics
    for ascites, 28
    and constipation, 59
    for dyspnea, 98
    for edema, 102
Diuril. *See* Chlorthiazide
Diversion, definition of, 266
Do not resuscitate order, definition of, 266
Doctor shopper, definition of, 266
Docusate sodium (Colace). *See also*
        Casanthrol and docusate sodium
    for bowel obstruction, 40
Dolophine. *See* Methadone
Dopamine antagonists, for nausea and
        vomiting, 181*t*
Double effect, principle of, 231
Dronabinol (Marinol)
    for anorexia, 18
    for nausea and vomiting, 181*t*
    in pain management, 189*t*
Drooling, 94
Droperidol (Inapsine)
    for nausea and vomiting, 182
    for terminal sedation, 233
Drug Abuse Warning Network, definition
        of, 266
Drug Enforcement Administration (DEA)
    definition of, 266
    and legal issues in pain management,
        170–171
Drugs, 259–263, 268–269. *See also*
        Medications
    definition of, 266
Drug toxicity, and delirium, 81
Dulcolax. *See* Bisacodyl
Durable power of attorney for health care
    definition of, 1
    family and, 112
Duraclon. *See* Clonidine
Duragesic. *See* Fentanyl
Dying, 71–75
    definition of, 71
    management of, 72–74
    manifestations of, 71–72
    pathophysiology/etiology of, 71
    physiology of, 19

Dysphagia, 93–95
    definition of, 93
    management of, 94
    manifestations of, 93–94
    pathophysiology/etiology of, 93
Dyspnea, 97–99
    definition of, 97
    during dying process, 73
    management of, 98
    manifestations of, 97–98
    pathophysiology/etiology of, 97

E

Edema, 101–103. *See also* Lymphedema
    definition of, 101
    management of, 102–103
    manifestations of, 101
    pathophysiology/etiology of, 101
Edmonton Comfort Assessment Form, 196
Edmonton Symptoms Assessment System, 196
Effexor. *See* Venlafaxine
Elase. *See* Fibrinolysin
Elavil. *See* Amitriptyline
Emesis, with bowel obstruction, 39
Emotional concerns, difficult articulation of, 203
End-of-life care
    definition of, 266
    resources on, 258
Enemas, for constipation, 60
Enteral nutrition support, 16–17
    contraindications to, 16–17
    indications for, 16
    problems in, troubleshooting, 17*t*
    starting, 17–18
Equianalgesic, definition of, 267
Erythropoietin
    for anemia, 10
    for asthenia, 32
    for dyspnea, 98
Esophageal dysphagia, 93–94
Essential oils, 52*t*
Estate of Henry James v. Hillhaven Corp., 173
Ethical conflict, prevention and resolution
        of, 256
Ethical directives, 107
Ethics, 105–109

definition of, 105
principle-based, 106, 106t–107t
promotion of, strategies for, 107–108
of terminal sedation, 231
Eutectic mixture of local anesthetic,
    definition of, 267
Evidence-based practice, resources on,
    258
Exercise, for edema, 102
Existential concerns, difficult articulation
    of, 203
Expectations, communication about, 49
Expectorants, for cough, 64

F

FACIT. *See* Functional Assessment of
    Chronic Illness Therapy
FACT-An. *See* Functional Assessment of
    Cancer Therapy-Anemia
Fairness approach, to ethics, 106
Famciclovir (Famvir), for zoster, 246
Family
    and advance directives, 1–2
    and bereavement, 35–37
    and caregiver burden, 43–45
    and communication, 47–49
    and complementary therapies, 51
    cultural awareness and, 67–69
    definition of, 267
    and dying process, 72–74
    fears of, 119
    and funeral planning, 127
    and grief, 130
    and home care, 137
    and hope, 144–145
    hospice care and, 148
    and isolation, 165
    optimal functioning of, strategies for,
        112–113
    outcomes with, 113
    psychologic support for, 203–204
    and voluntary refusal of food and
        fluids, 20
Family issues, 111–114
    definition of, 111
Famvir. *See* Famciclovir
Fatigue, 115–117
    definition of, 115
    management of, 116

manifestations of, 115–116
pathophysiology/etiology of, 115
Fear, 119–121
    of abandonment, 165, 205
    about home care, 138–139
    addressing, 119–120
    definition of, 119
    diminishing, strategies for, 120
    of pain, 185
Fecal incontinence collectors, 90
Feeding education, for dysphagia, 94
Fentanyl (Duragesic), 188t
    for neuropathic pain, 248
    for pain, 190
Ferrous sulfate. *See* Iron supplements
Fever, 123–125
    definition of, 123
    manifestations of, 123–125
    pathophysiology/etiology of, 123
Fibrinolysin (Elase), for skin lesions, 223
Fidelity, and ethics, 107t
Financial issues
    and caregiver burden, 43
    and funeral planning, 128
    and hospice care, 148
Flagyl. *See* Metronidazole
Fluconazole (Diflucan)
    for fungal infection, 152
    for xerostomia, 244
Fluids
    and edema, 102
    voluntary refusal of, 19–20
Fluoxetine (Prozac)
    for depression, 86t
    for neuropathic pain, 248
Foley catheter, 240
Food, voluntary refusal of, 19–20
Fullness, feelings of, management of, 14–15
Functional Assessment of Cancer Therapy-
    Anemia (FACT-An), 117
Functional Assessment of Chronic Illness
    Therapy (FACIT), 117
Funeral planning, 127–128
    definition of, 127
Fungal infections, treatment of, 152
Furosemide (Lasix)
    for ascites, 28
    for dyspnea, 98
    for edema, 102
Future care, communication about, 48

G

Gabapentin (Neurontin)
  for neuropathic pain, 247
  in pain management, 189*t*
  for seizures, 212
Gabitril. *See* Tiagabine
Gamma-aminobutyric acid agonists, for
    neuropathic pain, 250
Glycopyrrolate (Robinul)
  during dying process, 74
  for nausea and vomiting, 181*t*
Grief, 35–37, 129–131. *See also* Loss.
  definition of, 129
  time frame of, 129
  types of, 129–130

H

HADS. *See* Hospital Anxiety and Depres-
    sion Scale
Halcion. *See* Triazolam
Haloperidol (Haldol)
  for agitation, 6
  for anxiety, 25
  for delirium, 82
  for hiccups, 134
  for nausea and vomiting, 181*t*, 182
Harp, 55
Healing, definition of, 267
Health history, for travel, 235
Health Insurance Association of America,
    163
Hiccups, 133–135
  definition of, 133
  management of, 133–134
  manifestations of, 133
  pathophysiology/etiology of, 133
Holistic approach to care, 165
  and spirituality, 228
Home care. *See also* Hospice care
  advantages and disadvantages of, 138*f*
  and caregiver burden, 44
  versus hospital, 137–141
  insurance coverage for, 160
Hope, 143–146
  definition of, 143
  dimensions of, 143
  threats to, 144
Hopelessness, 143–145

Hospice care, 140, 147–150. *See also*
    Home care
  and caregivers, 44
  definition of, 147, 267
  insurance coverage for, 148, 159–160
Hospice Quality of Life Index, 196
Hospital Anxiety and Depression Scale
    (HADS), 87
Hospital care
  advantages and disadvantages of, 139*f*
  versus homecare, 137–141
Humidification, for cough, 64
Hyaluronidase (Wydase), for dehydration,
    78
Hydration
  for diarrhea, 90
  for fever, 124
Hydrazine sulfate, for anorexia, 18
Hydrocodone, for neuropathic pain, 248
Hydrogen peroxide, for pressure ulcers,
    223
Hydromorphone (Dilaudid), 188*t*
  for neuropathic pain, 248
  for pain, 190
Hydrotherapy, 52
Hydroxyzine hydrochloride (Atarax), for
    pruritus, 200
Hyoscyamine butylbromide (Levsin)
  for bowel obstruction, 40
  during dying process, 74
  for nausea and vomiting, 181*t*
Hyperalgesia, definition of, 267
Hypercalcemia, and nausea, 180
Hypnotics, for insomnia, 156
Hypodermoclysis
  for agitation, 6
  for dehydration, 78
Hyponatremia, in SIADH, 102

I

IASP. *See* International Association for the
    Study of Pain
Ibuprofen (Motrin), for fever, 124
Illegal drug/narcotic, definition of, 267
Imipramine (Tofranil), for depression, 86*t*
Inapsine. *See* Droperidol
Infection, 151–154
  definition of, 151
  management of, 152–153

manifestations of, 151
pathophysiology/etiology of, 151
Informed consent
for sedation, 232
in voluntary refusal of food and fluids,
20
Inpatient care
in hospice, 148
insurance coverage for, 161
Insomnia, 155–157
definition of, 155
management of, 156–157
manifestations of, 155–156
pathophysiology/etiology of, 155
Insurance, 159–164
coverage limits, 161–162
and hospice care, 148, 159–160
strategies for, 162
Interdisciplinary care, in hospice care, 147
Interferons, and cachexia, 13
Interleukins, and cachexia, 13
Intermittent self-catheterization (ISC),
240
International Association for the Study of
Pain (IASP), 185
Intraperitoneal therapy, for ascites, 29
Intrathecal pumps (IPs), for neuropathic
pain, 251
Invasive treatments, for neuropathic pain,
250–251
Ipratropium (Atrovent), for dyspnea, 98
IPs. *See* Intrathecal pumps
Iron supplements
for anemia, 9–10
and constipation, 59
for fatigue, 116
and nausea, 179
Irrigation, for pressure ulcers, 223
ISC. *See* Intermittent self-catheterization
Isolation, 165–168
definition of, 165
prevention of, strategies for, 166–167
Isoproterenol (Isuprel), for dyspnea, 98

J

Joint Commission on Accreditation of
Healthcare Organizations
(JCAHO), 169, 173
Justice, and ethics, 106, 107*t*

K

Keflex. *See* Cephalexin
Keppra. *See* Levetiracetam
Klonopin. *See* Clonazepam

L

Lactulose (Chronulac), for constipation, 60
Lamotrigine (Lamictal)
for neuropathic pain, 247
in pain management, 189*t*
Lasix. *See* Furosemide
Lavender *(Lavandula angustifolia)* oil, 52*t*
Legal issues, in pain management, 169–
173
LeVeen catheter, for ascites, 29
Levetiracetam (Keppra), for neuropathic
pain, 247
Levorphanol, for neuropathic pain, 248
Levsin. *See* Hyoscyamine butylbromide
Lidocaine. *See* Xylocaine
Lioresal. *See* Baclofen
Lithium, and delirium, 81
Living will, definition of, 1
Loading dose, definition of, 267
Local analgesics, for neuropathic pain, 248–
249
Long-term care, insurance coverage for, 161
Loop diuretics, for ascites, 28
Lorazepam (Ativan)
for anxiety, 24
for nausea and vomiting, 181*t*, 182
for neuropathic pain, 250
for seizures, 212
for terminal sedation, 233
Loss. *See also* Grief
psychologic support for, 205
Lubrication, for intercourse, 216–217
Lymphedema, 175–177. *See also* Edema
definition of, 175
management of, 175–176
manifestations of, 175
pathophysiology/etiology of, 175

M

Maalox-Plus. *See* Simethicone
Macrodantin. *See* Nitrofurantoin
Maintenance dose, definition of, 267

Malignant cutaneous wounds
definition of, 221
management of, 222–225
pathophysiology/etiology of, 221
staging of, 222
Malpractice, 172
Marcaine. *See* Bupivicaine
Marinol. *See* Dronabinol
Massage
with aromatherapy, 52–53
for lymphedema, 176
Measurement instruments
for ascites, 30
for cachexia, 21
for depression, 87–88
for fatigue, 117
for insomnia, 157
for lymphedema, 177
for pain, 191
in palliative care, 196–197
for quality of life, 209
resources on, 257
Medicaid Waiver Program, 44–45
Medicare
hospice benefit, 159–160
information on, 163
skilled nursing facility coverage, 161
Medications. *See also* Drugs
during dying process, 72–73
for travel, 236
Medrol. *See* Methylprednisone
Megastrol acetate (Megace)
for anorexia, 19
for asthenia, 32
Melatonin, for insomnia, 157
Metaproterenol (Alupent), for dyspnea, 98
Methadone (Dolophine), 188*t*
for cough, 64
for neuropathic pain, 248
for pain, 190
Methylphenidate (Ritalin)
for asthenia, 32
for depression, 86, 86*t*, 87
Methylprednisone (Medrol)
for dyspnea, 98
in pain management, 190
Metoclopramide (Reglan)
for bowel obstruction, 40
for hiccups, 134
for nausea and vomiting, 181*t*, 182

Metronidazole (Flagyl), for skin lesions, 224
Mexiletine (Mexitil)
for neuropathic pain, 248–249
for pain, 190
in pain management, 189*t*
Micronutrient deficiencies, enteral feeding and, 18
Midazolam (Versed)
for delirium, 82
for hiccups, 134
for seizures, 212
for terminal sedation, 233
Milk of magnesia, for constipation, 60
Mirtazapine (Remeron), for depression, 86*t*
Missoula-Vitas Quality of Life Index, 196
Mixed opiate agonist-antagonist, definition of, 267
Moisturizers, for pruritus, 200
Morphine, 188*t*
for dyspnea, 98
for neuropathic pain, 247–248
for pain, 190
Motrin. *See* Ibuprofen
Mourning, 35–37
elements of, 129
grief and, 129–131
optimal, 36
Mouth, sore, management of, 15
Multidimensional approach, and quality of life, 208
Music therapy, 54–55
Mycostatin. *See* Nystatin

N

Narcotics. *See also* Opiates
for cough, 64
definition of, 267
Nardostachys jatamansi (spikenard), 52*t*
National Viatical Association, 163
Nausea, 179–183
with bowel obstruction, 39
definition of, 179
management of, 15–16, 180–182
manifestations of, 180
pain management and, 190
pathophysiology/etiology of, 179
Nearing death awareness, 72–73

Neostigmine methylsulfate (Prostigmin),
for dysphagia, 94
Neurontin. *See* Gabapentin
Neuropathic pain
analgesic stepladder for, 251
definition of, 268
management of, 247–253
manifestations of, 186
Nifedipine (Procardia), for hiccups, 134
Nitrofurantoin (Macrodantin), for infection, 152
Nociceptive pain, 185–186
Nonmaleficence, and ethics, 106*t*
Nonsteroidal anti-inflammatory drugs (NSAIDs)
definition of, 267
and nausea, 179
for neuropathic pain, 250
for pain, 187
Norpramin. *See* Desipramine
Nortriptyline (Pamelor)
for depression, 86*t*
for neuropathic pain, 248
in pain management, 189*t*
NSAIDs. *See* Nonsteroidal anti-inflammatory drugs
Nursing home care, 139–140
Medicare hospice benefit and, 160
Nutrition, for fatigue, 116
Nutritional support, 13–22
Nystatin (Mycostatin)
for dysphagia, 94
for xerostomia, 244

O

Octreotide (Sandostatin)
for ascites, 29
for bowel obstruction, 40
Olanzapine (Zyprexa)
for agitation, 6
for delirium, 82
for nausea and vomiting, 181*t*
Ondansetron (Zofran), for nausea and vomiting, 181*t*, 182
Opiate(s)
for anxiety, 25
for bowel obstruction, 40
and constipation, 59
definition of, 267

for dysphagia, 94
for dyspnea, 98
legal issues with, 169–173
and nausea, 179
for neuropathic pain, 247–248
for severe pain, 188–189
for terminal sedation, 233
Opiate receptors, definition of, 267
Opiate rotation, 248
Opiate titration, 248
Oropharyngeal dysphagia, 93
Oxcarbazepine (Trileptal), for neuropathic pain, 247
Oxycodone, 188*t*
for neuropathic pain, 248
Oxygen
for anemia, 10
for anxiety, 25
for cough, 64
for dyspnea, 98

P

Pain, 185–192. *See also* Neuropathic pain
acute, definition of, 268
assessment and evaluation of, 186
breakthrough, 185, 188
chronic, definition of, 266
crescendo, 81
definition of, 185, 267
manifestations of, 185–186
pathophysiology/etiology of, 185
somatic, manifestations of, 185–186
Pain affect, definition of, 268
Pain management, 186–190
barriers to, 187
goals of, 186–187
legal issues in, 169–173
of neuropathic pain, 247–253
resources on, 257
side effects of, 190
by source of pain, 187*t*
Palliative care, 193–197
definition of, 193, 268
focus of, 194
insurance coverage for, 161
levels of, 194
promotion of, strategies for, 194–195
as specialty, 193
Palliative Care Outcome Scale (POS), 196

Pamelor. *See* Nortriptyline
Pamidronate (Aredia)
   for pain, 190
   in pain management, 189*t*
Papain urea (Accuzyme), for skin lesions, 223
Paracentesis, for ascites, 28–29
Parenteral nutrition support, 18
Paroxetine (Paxil)
   for depression, 86*t*
   for neuropathic pain, 248
Patient Self-Determination Act (PSDA), 2
Paxil. *See* Paroxetine
Peer review, definition of, 268
Pemoline. *See* Cylert
Peppermint water, for hiccups, 134
Periactin. *See* Cyproheptadine hydrochloride
Peri-Colace. *See* Casanthrol and docusate sodium
Peritoneovenous shunts, for ascites, 29
Pharmaceutical Research and Manufactureres Association of America, 163
Pharyngitis, and dysphagia, 94
Phenazopyridine (Pyridium), for infection, 152
Phenergan. *See* Promethazine
Phenobarbital
   for seizures, 212
   for terminal sedation, 233
Phenothiazines
   for anxiety, 25
   and constipation, 59
   for dyspnea, 98
   for nausea and vomiting, 181*t*
Phenytoin (Dilantin)
   for hiccups, 134
   for seizures, 212
Physical dependence, definition of, 268
Physical modalities, definition of, 268
Physiotherapy, complex decongestive, for lymphedema, 176
Pilocarpine (Salagen)
   for dysphagia, 94
   for xerostomia, 244
Piper Fatigue Scale, 117
Pneumocystis carinii infection, 152
POS. *See* Palliative Care Outcome Scale
Povidone iodine, for pressure ulcers, 223

PQRST mnemonic, 186
Prednisone (Deltasone)
   for asthenia, 32
   for dyspnea, 98
   in pain management, 189*t*, 190
Pressure ulcers, 221–226
   definition of, 221
   management of, 222–225
   manifestations of, 221–222
   pathophysiology/etiology of, 221
   prevention of, 223
   staging of, 222
Prime-MD Mood Module, 87
Principle-based ethics, 106, 106*t*–107*t*
Procardia. *See* Nifedipine
Prochlorperazine (Compazine)
   for bowel obstruction, 40
   for nausea and vomiting, 181*t*
Program of All-Inclusive Care of the Elderly, 161
Promethazine (Phenergan), for nausea and vomiting, 181*t*
Prostigmin. *See* Neostigmine methylsulfate
Proventil. *See* Albuterol
Prozac. *See* Fluoxetine
Pruritus, 199–201
   definition of, 199
   management of, 199–200
   manifestations of, 199
   pathophysiology/etiology of, 199
PSDA. *See* Patient Self-Determination Act
Pseudoaddiction, definition of, 268
Psychologic support, 203–206
   definition of, 203
   for fatigue, 116
   strategies for, 203–205
Psychostimulants, 86, 86*t*
   and insomnia, 155
Psyllium products, for diarrhea, 90
Pyridium. *See* Phenazopyridine

Q

Quality of life (QOL), 207–209
   definition of, 207
   individual's definition of, 208
   maintenance of, strategies for, 208
Questran. *See* Cholestyramine
Quetiapine (Seroquel), for agitation, 6
Quinidine, and delirium, 81

R

Radiation therapy
and anemia, 9
for dyspnea, 98
for malignant cutaneous wounds, 223
Recombinant growth hormone, for
anorexia, 19
Reglan. *See* Metoclopramide
Regulatory complaint, definition of, 268
Reiki, 53–54
Relaxation, and sexual intercourse, 217
Remeron. *See* Mirtazapine
Respiration, during dying process, 74
Respiratory tract infection, treatment of,
152
Respite care
definition of, 268
in hospice, 148–149
Restlessness, versus spiritual need, 227
Restoril. *See* Temazepam
Rights approach, to ethics, 106
Risperidone (Risperdal)
for agitation, 6
for delirium, 82
Ritalin. *See* Methylphenidate
Robinul. *See* Glycopyrrolate
Routine care, in hospice, 148

S

Sadness, versus depression, 85–86
Salagen. *See* Pilocarpine
Saliva, 243
Sandostatin. *See* Octreotide
Santyl. *See* Collagenase
Satiety, early, management of, 14–15
Schedule I drugs, definition of, 268
Schedule II drugs, definition of, 268–269
Schedule III drugs, definition of, 269
Schedule IV drugs, definition of, 269
Schedule V drugs, definition of, 269
Scientific culture, 68
Scopolamine, for dyspnea, 98
Scopolamine hydrobromide, for bowel
obstruction, 40
Scopolamine transdermal patch
(Transderm-Scop)
during dying process, 74
for nausea and vomiting, 181*t*

SCSs. *See* Spinal cord stimulators
Sedation
pain management and, 190
terminal, 231–234
Seizures, 211–213
definition of, 211
management of, 211–212
manifestations of, 211
pathophysiology/etiology of, 211
Selective serotonin reuptake inhibitors
(SSRIs), 86, 86*t*
for neuropathic pain, 248
Self
loss of, 205
offering of, 204
therapeutic use of, 48
Self-determination, and ethics, 106*t*
Senior day care, 45
Senior services, 45
Senna (Senokot), for constipation, 60
Seroquel. *See* Quetiapine
Sertraline (Zoloft), for depression, 86*t*
Sexuality, 215–219
definition of, 215
expressions of, facilitating, strategies
for, 216–218
problems with, manifestations of, 216
Shingles, 245–246
SIADH. *See* Antidiuretic hormone,
inappropriate secretion of
Sildenafil (Viagra), 217–218
Simethicone (Maalox-Plus), for hiccups,
134
Skin care
for diarrhea, 90
for edema, 102
with pruritus, 199–200
Skin lesions, 221–226
Sleep diary, 157
Sleep disturbances, 155–157
Smell, alterations in, management of, 15
Sodium hypochlorite, for pressure ulcers,
223
Sodium restriction, for ascites, 28
Somatic pain, manifestations of, 185–186
Somatostatin analog, for bowel obstruction,
40
Sorbitol, for constipation, 60
Spikenard *(Nardostachys jatamansi)* oil,
52*t*

Spinal cord stimulators (SCSs), for neuropathic pain, 251
Spiritual coping, indications of, 228
Spiritual distress, manifestations of, 228
Spirituality, 227–230
    definition of, 227
    facilitation of, strategies for, 228–229
    and fear, 120
    hope and, 143
Spiritual needs, individuality of, 227
Spironolactone (Aldactone)
    for ascites, 28
    for dyspnea, 98
    for edema, 102
Spritzer, for aromatherapy, 53
SSRIs. *See* Selective serotonin reuptake inhibitors
State medical boards, and legal issues in pain management, 171–172
Status epilepticus, definition of, 211
Steroids
    and insomnia, 155
    for neuropathic pain, 250
    for pruritus, 200
Stomatitis, and dysphagia, 94
Suctioning, for cough, 64
Suffering, definition of, 269
Sundown syndrome, 81
Support, for bereavement, 36
Suppositories
    for constipation, 60
    contraindications for, 124
    during dying process, 73
    for nausea and vomiting, 182
Symptom control, versus maintaining cognitive function, 207

T

Tagamet. *See* Cimetidine
Takata, Hawayo, 54
Taste, alterations in, management of, 15
TCAs. *See* Tricyclic antidepressants
Technology, life-prolonging, unnecessary, and palliative care, 193
Tegretol. *See* Carbamazepine
Temazepam (Restoril), for insomnia, 156
Tenckhoff catheter, for ascites, 29
Terminal illness, definition of, 269
Terminal phase, assessment of, 195

Terminal sedation, 231–234
    definition of, 231
    indications for, 231–232
    management of, 232–233
    pathophysiology/etiology of, 231
Tessalon Perles. *See* Benzonatate
Theophylline (Theo-Dur), for dyspnea, 98
Therapeutic communication, 47–50
Therapeutic touch (TT), 53
Thorazine. *See* Chlorpromazine
Throat, sore, management of, 15
Tiagabine (Gabitril), for neuropathic pain, 247
Tigan. *See* Trimethobenzamide
Titrate, definition of, 269
Tizanidine (Zanaflex), for neuropathic pain, 249
Tofranil. *See* Imipramine
Tolerance, definition of, 269
Toolkit of Instruments to Measure Care at the End of Life, 196–197
Topical analgesics, for neuropathic pain, 248–249
Tramadol, 188*t*
Transcutaneous electrical nerve stimulation, definition of, 269
Transderm-Scop. *See* Scopolamine transdermal patch
Tranxene. *See* Chlorazepate
Travel, 235–237
    management of, 235–236
Treatment, aggressive, choice to discontinue, 207
Triazolam (Halcion)
    for insomnia, 156
    for terminal sedation, 233
Tricyclic antidepressants (TCAs), 86, 86*t*
    for neuropathic pain, 248
    in pain management, 189–190, 189*t*
    for pruritus, 200
Trigeminal neuralgia, 247
Trileptal. *See* Oxcarbazepine
Trimethobenzamide (Tigan), for nausea and vomiting, 181*t*
Trimethoprim/sulfamethoxazole (Bactrim), for infection, 152
TT. *See* Therapeutic touch
Tumor necrosis factor, and cachexia, 13
Tylenol. *See* Acetaminophen

U

Uncomplicated grief, 130
Unfinished business
    and grief, 129
    isolation and, 166
Urea, for edema, 102
Urecholine. *See* Bethanechol
Urinary elimination, 239–241
    definition of, 239
Urinary problems
    during dying process, 73
    management of, 239–240
    manifestations of, 239
    pathophysiology/etiology of, 239
Urinary tract infection, treatment of, 152
Usui, Mikao, 54
Utilitarian approach, to ethics, 106

V

Valacyclovir (Valtrex), for zoster, 246
Valerian root extract, for insomnia, 157
Valium. *See* Diazepam
Valproic acid (Depakene), for seizures, 212
Valtrex. *See* Valacyclovir
Varicella zoster virus (VZV), 245–246
Venlafaxine (Effexor), for neuropathic pain,
    248
Versed. *See* Midazolam
Viagra. *See* Sildenafil
Virtue approach, to ethics, 106
Visceral pain, manifestations of, 186
Vomiting, 179–183
    with bowel obstruction, 39
    definition of, 179
    management of, 15–16, 180–182
    manifestations of, 180
    pathophysiology/etiology of, 179
VZV. *See Varicella zoster* virus

W

Water restriction, for ascites, 28
Weakness. *See* Asthenia

Well-being, promoting, 255–256
Wydase. *See* Hyaluronidase

X

Xanax. *See* Alprazolam
Xerostomia, 243–244
    definition of, 243
    and dysphagia, 94
    management of, 243–244
    manifestations of, 243
    pathophysiology/etiology of, 243
Xylocaine (Lidocaine)
    for cough, 64
    for dysphagia, 94
    for neuropathic pain, 249

Y

Yeast infections
    oil-based lubricants and, 217
    treatment of, 152

Z

Zanaflex. *See* Tizanidine
Zithromax. *See* Azithromycin
Zofran. *See* Ondansetron
Zoloft. *See* Sertraline
Zolpidem (Ambien), for insomnia, 156
Zonasamide (Zonegran), for neuropathic
    pain, 247
Zoster, 245–246
    definition of, 245
    management of, 245–246
    manifestations of, 245
    pathophysiology/etiology of, 245
Zostrix. *See* Capsaicin
Zovirax. *See* Acyclovir
Zyprexa. *See* Olanzapine